THE CAFFEINE DIET

sipping your way to slim

by

Dr. Jeffry Weiss

A WORD OF CAUTION

Always notify your family doctor whenever embarking on a new diet. Have your vitals checked and tell him your diet plans. Make it clear that you will only be consuming 100 mg. of caffeine at a time: 5-6 times per day. But don't expect a ringing endorsement. Doctors are not trained in diet/nutritional matters. Your doctor will tell you that caffeine raises blood pressure, when, in fact, caffeine lowers blood pressure by flushing the kidneys. (That and other myths will be debunked in the body of the text).

When you understand the reasons why you are overweight and why every diet and exercise program (not you!) has failed, you will be set free by *The Caffeine Diet* and cure yourself of being a slave to food, hunger, bingeing, cravings, deprivation, and obesity once and for all.

It is essential to read this book to understand how caffeine works its magic and how to use caffeine to your maximum advantage. Do not simply start taking caffeine tablets or drinking coffee. You must follow the directions carefully to gain the maximum benefits and avoid the pitfalls.

On the Caffeine Diet you will experience a total reversal of the causes and weaknesses that currently rule your life, the factors that stop you from making wise food choices, and rob you of your health and self-esteem. There are no charts, tables, list, or monstrous exercise regime. You will not have to rely willpower or change your lifestyle. This is fundamental to our program. We, as a people, do not have the time or flexibility to make our lives over. And you won't have to on the Caffeine Diet.

OUR PROMISE

The information and direction provided herein will empower you to take control of not only your appetite but your life. You will reach your ideal weight (and maintain that), and regain your health and your self-esteem.

Make no mistake, while the premise is quite simple, the results are no less than amazing. Have faith. I know that you have gotten your hopes up before, and that even with all your willpower, you have failed. Of course you failed, you were relying on information that was thirty years old, left-over facts that were re-heated and served up once again after never having worked in the first place. On the Caffeine Diet you will have the metabolism of a thin person. When you have the correct metabolism, you cannot fail. It's the only thing that's been holding you back.

Nothing new has been said in regards to diet in three decades. And while "professionals" argue over the percentage of fats, protein, and carbohydrates in the diet, obesity rates have gone from 10% of the population to 50% in just 50 years.

The purveyors of magic elixirs, severely restricted calorie diets, blood type diets, low-carb diets, high-protein diets have no clue as to why people cannot lose weight and keep it off, or how to end that addiction. Their advice and findings are based on limited research and faulty logic.

On the Caffeine Diet you will learn how and when to use caffeine to its maximum advantage. Further, with your appetite under control, we will provide you with a dietary program based on 6 ½ million years of evolution, not three decades of antidotal evidence.

Until now, you have relied on health care experts who were anything but, and sent off on a wrong direction, by yourself, with incorrect information, no support, and no inspiration. You will not fail on this program. It is impossible to fail when you duplicate the metabolism of a thin person and the dietary guidelines followed by the healthiest people in the world. And we will show you who they are and what they eat and how they live.

Be prepared to take out that size six dress from the back of your closet, or those size thirty-two waist pants from mothballs. Don't give up even if you have failed many times in the past. Begin by reading this book and get on the program today. I can assure you that dependence on food as your primary source of euphoria is a thing of the past.

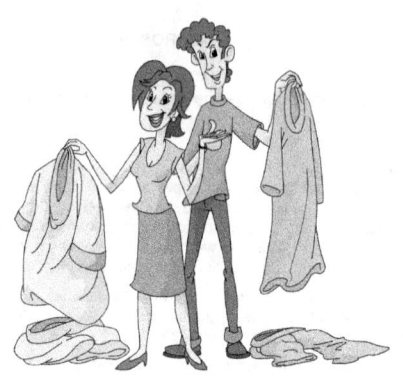

TABLE OF CONTENTS

Chapter	Page

INTRO: WHY DIETS DO NOT WORK

Caffeine is the secret of health and long life that Ponce De Leon searched for – Dr. Jeffry Weiss

Conventional Diets

It is impossible to lose weight by going on a conventional diet. As soon as you begin to lose weight, the body thinks you are in starvation mode and slows down the metabolic rate. A person who maintained a steady weight while eating 2400 calories, and then goes on a failed diet, will gain weight eating only 1200 calories! Most people, dependent on diet alone, would have to consume eight hundred calories per day, or less, to lose weight.

It is impossible to get enough essential vitamins and minerals in eight hundred calories to maintain a healthy, functional immune system. A plethora of diseases would follow. One cannot consume enough calcium and magnesium to build bone and thereby almost assuredly would undergo osteoporosis. Food cravings and bingeing would overwhelm even the strongest resolve. Without certain nutrients, anxiety and depression are assured.

Your Metabolic Rate

You might ask, "Why is our metabolic rate is so low now that we can't possibly succeed on a diet? What has changed so drastically in the last fifty years to precipitate obesity rates to go from 10% of the population in 1950 to 50% of the population in 2007?" That is a fair question. The answer is fluoridation.

Fluoride

Fluoridation of our water supply is the key contributor to the greatly increased rate of obesity in the past 50 years. It is no coincidence that fluoridation of our water supply began in 1950, when only one in ten people were obese. Today, 50 years after

fluoridation began, obesity rates have reached 50%** of the population (** Using 1950's standards, which have been relaxed to make us seem less fat).

Fluoridation of our water supplies significantly inhibits DNA synthesis and repair enzymes. Even as little as 1 part per million of fluoride inhibits DNA repair activity by 50%. Animal studies found that in 1 part per million, fluoride has caused chromosome damage.

Thyroid hormones rely on iodine, which is in the same group of four elements as fluorine. Fluorine displaces iodine in the body, which leads to serious problems with the thyroid gland. Children can be particularly affected if their mother was short of iodine during pregnancy.

Fluoridation affects thyroid function. The thyroid gland has a major role in controlling the metabolic rate. Fluoride slows down that rate, thereby burning fewer calories during the day. Fluoridation of our water supply is a key contributor to the greatly increased rate of obesity in the past 50 years. It is no coincidence that fluoridation of our water supply began in 1950, when only one in ten people were obese. Today, 50 years after fluoridation began, one in two people are obese.

Fluoridation is the generic name for the process of treating our water supplies. Technically the process is Aluminum fluoridation. Yes, aluminum, as in one of the primary causes of Alzheimer's disease! Autopsies of the brains of people who have died due to Alzheimer's disease showed a direct causal relationship between the absorption of aluminum (either through food or environmental exposure) and the disease. To reach the brain, aluminum must pass the blood-brain barrier, an elaborate structure that filters the blood before it reaches this vital organ. Elemental aluminum does not readily pass through this barrier, but certain aluminum compounds, such as aluminum fluoride, do. Many municipal water supplies are treated with both aluminum sulfate and aluminum fluoride, and these two chemicals readily combine with each other in the blood. Moreover, aluminum fluoride, once formed, is very poorly excreted in the urine.

The obesity epidemic that is plaguing the US, the UK and other industrialized countries is unequivocally linked to fluoride in drinking water. Dr Barry Durrant-Peatfield says that "there is no doubt that fluoride is enzyme disruptive and one thing it affects is thyroid hormones", adding that "People end up with an under-activity of the thyroid gland." And children may be particularly susceptible to obesity if their mothers drank fluoridated water while pregnant.

Exactly how does the environment affect the thyroid?

We now have substantial research to demonstrate that environmental chemicals have a direct impact on the thyroid gland. It's clear that PCBs and other industrial petrochemical toxins can lower thyroid function, as well as other pollutants such as chlorine, bromide, and fluoride. Almost all these elements and dangers reach us via our water supply. And the primary contributor to an under-active thyroid is fluoride.

Since the thyroid produces hormones that manage your metabolism, anything that affects your thyroid will ultimately affect your metabolism. In fact, there's evidence that toxins boost the excretion of thyroid hormones, leaving you with less of this hormone to control your metabolism - and a decreased ability to burn fat. The truth is your thyroid plays a huge role in weight control, and in determining your metabolic rate.

The question is not if, but how much is today's obesity epidemic linked to the harmful effects of environmental toxins on metabolism. I've seen so many patients struggle with their weight, only to have the pounds melt off when we addressed their thyroid problems.

Now here is the most important question. How do we address those thyroid problems? Allopathic medicine (mainstream medicine) uses pharmaceutical drugs to treat thyroid malfunction. These drugs have serious side effects and do not boost the metabolic rates to optimal levels and hold it there all day. Pharmaceutical meds are one size, fits all. Further, these drugs are known to produce anxiety, depression, debilitating migraine headaches, fuzzy thinking, memory problems, etc. They are not tailored to individual needs or individual metabolisms, or changes to metabolism that happen over time. Many doctors can miss the subtle signs of thyroid problems, and conventional medicine often treats low thyroid function with inadequate, one-size-fits-all drugs like Synthroid. Thyroid dysfunction requires you to become an active partner in your care.

Following is a list of the symptoms of a low thyroid function:

Fatigue
Sluggishness
Trouble Getting up in the Morning
Depression
Dry Skin
Dry Hair
Constipation
Fluid Retention
Menstrual Problems And Pms
Hair Loss
Cracked or Chipping Fingernails
Low Sex Drive
Weight Gain
Muscle Aches
Cramps

Yes, a lot of those symptoms are pretty common and vague - which is one reason why thyroid dysfunction often goes undetected.

Other factors that can affect thyroid deficiencies

Now let's talk about some of those other factors. For example, food allergies, like sensitivities to gluten and other foods, also negatively affect thyroid function - and are frequently undiagnosed. Likewise, deficiencies in nutrients important to good thyroid function - like selenium, zinc, omega-3 fatty acids, iodine and tyrosine - can also trigger thyroid problems. We will review these and more in the following chapters. With all of these factors that can affect your thyroid, it's clear that we need a new approach to the diagnosis and treatment of thyroid disease in order to regain control of our appetites and maintain a healthy, attractive, desired weight.

There's no doubt that thyroid disease is on the rise. From the research I've reviewed and the patients I've seen in the last 20 years, it's clear to me that the thyroid gland is sensitive to many different influences - your diet, your lifestyle, and the world around you.

So, it's not surprising that as we eat more toxic foods and are increasingly exposed to pollution, petrochemical and industrial wastes, and heavy metals that thyroid problems have skyrocketed. In fact, more than 80% of women and men in the United States have thyroid dysfunctions - and half of them don't even know it!

Correcting a dysfunctional thyroid

Know that the problem can be fixed . . . simply. By following the program here you can get your thyroid working properly, keep your weight under control, and start feeling better today. And you will be in total control of your thyroid, metabolism, and weight loss goals. On my program I will teach you how you can ignite the fat burning code hidden in your own DNA.

You cannot eliminate all external or internal causes of an under active thyroid. What you can do is eliminate the most invasive and prevalent, and then follow the (very) simple program presented here.

Tap water can make you fat

Medical experts confirm that tap water can make people fat and is fuelling rising obesity levels. For the past fifty years, fluoride has been pumped into our tap water to help keep teeth healthy. And now major medical institutions confirm that the toxin causes worrying health side-effects including hypothyroidism, a medical disorder affecting the thyroid gland which controls weight gain.

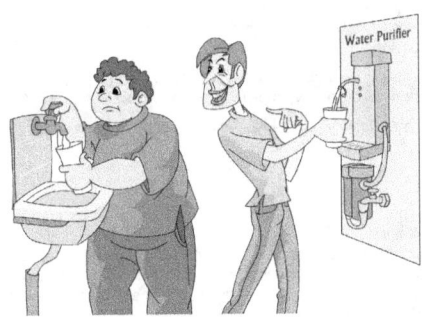

Can't you simply stop drinking tap water? It's not that simple. Even if you have a good filtration system for the drinking water in your home you still absorb the equivalent of eight 8 ounce glasses of water every time you take a shower. Further, that would still not address the other toxins in our environment that affect the thyroid or water drank outside the home. And no, bottled water - unless it employs activated charcoal, reverse osmosis and distillation – is beneficial.

The four ways to lose weight

In the face of this research, what can we do? First, let's be clear about the ways there are to lose weight. For decades, doctors and health care professionals have been telling people that there are only two ways to lose weight: eat fewer calories and exercise more. Well there are, in fact, four ways to lose weight, not two.

When people are confronted by those two unsuccessful ways, the choice for most is neither, and they give up before even starting. The four ways are:

1) Exercise
2) Eat fewer calories
3) Boost metabolic rate which raises
   core temperature, causing more calories to be burned (thermogensis)
4) Promote fat burning (lipolysis), predominately from the abnormal stores of fat

The answers to all our questions

Now, what if there were a substance that boosted the metabolic rate to pre-1950s level, that was both thermogenic and lipolytic? And what if this substance also triggered the release of a hormone (CCK) that signaled the brain to shut down the eating process, protected against Alzheimer's disease, Parkinson's disease, liver disease, and breast cancer, improved learning and retention, sped up reaction time (think driving on crowded roads), reduced the risk of diabetes by 30%, enabled one to work out 20% longer and more intensely, think more cogently and fluently, multi-task more effectively, feel happier (moderate depression), be more self-confident, eat less, and even act as a powerful antioxidant?

How does that sound? It sounds like coffee! And there's still more. Caffeine enhances the effects of serotonin, which, as you know, improves mood. Caffeine tells your cells to ignore the chemical adenosine, which promotes sleep, and it increases dopamine, which lifts mood and has been shown to prevent depression.

Caffeine improves sleep quality as well as overcomes fatigue, combats jet lag, elevates intelligence and memory, enhances creativity, improves mood and dispels

Boredom while increasing sociability, and slows aging while counteracting disease. Indeed, caffeine appears as an elixir of life to the informed user.

What now?

So, how can one use caffeine to its maximum advantage? In the course of this book we will address every step of the program and answer any questions and concerns that you might have. I do not wish to disparage other health care provides. Yet allopathic (MDs) doctors receive only one course in nutrition during their entire careers. They are taught to heal the sick, not prevent people from getting sick. I have studied diet and nutrition for over 40 years; that does not qualify me to do brain surgery.

If you have the same metabolic rate as a thin person, then you can follow a healthy eating plan (not a diet!), which will be outlined for you in detail later in this book, and lose the weight. With this program you will get thin and stay thin. There will be no dieting. As we have alluded to, diets simply do not work in the long run.

The dangers of following a conventional diet

Fat is stored in three areas of the body. First, structural fat around the joints and organs; second, normal fat reserves throughout the entire body; and third, abnormal fat reserves, which are known as the "problem areas. In women, these problem areas generally include the hips, thighs, buttocks, waist, stomach, and behind the upper arms; in men, the upper chest, back, neck, waist, and stomach. These abnormal fat reserves (the problem areas) are never released no matter how few calories you eat. The essential fat is the last to go on regular diets, and will only be released after all the normal fat reserves are exhausted. These reserves are a survival mechanism and will only be released after ninety days of starvation; as a last resort so that the person does not die.

On conventional diets the weight you lose is never the fat in the problem areas. You actually lose water, structural fat, and muscle. The body stores essential fat in what is, for us, the problem areas. The weight that is stored in the problem areas is virtually impossible to lose under normal circumstances.

On the Caffeine Diet you will lose the abnormal fat. You will have no food cravings and you will not feel deprived. You will not need willpower. Most importantly, you will lose very little, if any, structural fat and muscle. This means your body will be reshaped. It will look as if you have had liposuction. You will not lose the structural fat that you need for good health.

The limitations of Exercise

Exercise is a very important part of a healthy life style. Although exercise is encouraged, you do not need to exercise to attain results. Notice, I say "attain results." You will attain quicker and more impressive results if you do exercise. I have gone to the gym since I was a kid and continue to this day. Exercise triggers the release of endorphins which improve mood, boosts the immune system, bring on a euphoric state, and burns calories. I fully support all forms of exercise. However, you could exercise two hours a day along with dieting and still not lose the weight. Why? It just does not burn enough calories. Eat lunch at a fast food establishment: a cheese burger, fries, and a soda (2,000 calories approx.). Okay. How long would you have to walk (at a brisk pace) to burn off these calories? 10 minutes? Half hour? One hour? Two hours? Not even close. The answer is 7 1/3 hours (assuming your weigh 160 lbs.).

You need to exercise for all of the aforementioned reasons, but you can't rely simply on that. It will not work. You need to increase the metabolic rate: the rate at which the body, of its own accord, burns fat.

Calories Burned Per Hour *

Weight (lbs)	3mph	3.5 mph	4mph	4.5 mph	5mph
100	162	181	201	306	413
120	195	218	241	367	496
140	228	254	281	429	578
160	260	291	322	490	661
180	293	327	362	552	744
200	326	364	402	613	827

*Calories burned per hour by walking on a level surface without hand weights

Calories Burned Per Hour *

Weight (lbs)	Flat surface	5 % incline	10 % incline
100	162	229	296
110	179	252	326
120	195	275	355
130	212	298	385
140	228	321	141
150	244	345	445
160	260	367	474
170	276	389	503
180	293	413	533
190	309	435	562
200	326	459	593

* Calorie Expenditure per Hour While Walking, with Incline   Calories burned per hour Walking 3 miles per hour nearly doubles with a 10 percent incline.

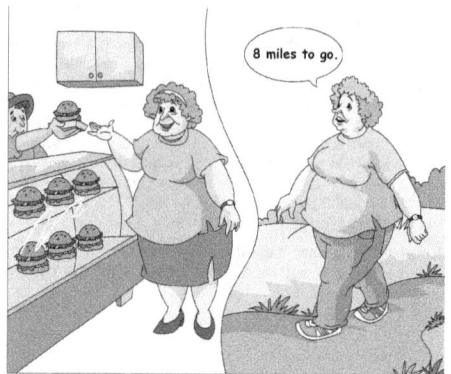

Is obesity genetic?

Why should I do all the work if obesity is genetic? There's nothing I can do that will ever make me thin. Well, if it is, you're off the hook . . . right? Wrong. It's not!

So, can I prove that obesity is habitual, not genetic?

You bet I can. New research shows that mothers-to-be can reduce the risk that their babies will develop obesity, high blood pressure, heart disease, and diabetes by simply monitoring their own diet during (not in the months and years before pregnancy – which would do even more to protect the unborn child from the afore-mentioned aliments). A recent study from the National Birth Defect Prevention Study found that a mother's nutrition and exercise patterns during pregnancy influence the long-term health of the baby by shaping the baby's metabolism. Metabolism includes everything that allows your body to turn food into energy: from the organ systems that process food and waste, to the energy-producing chemical reactions that take place inside every cell.

A mother's body influences her baby's metabolism in many levels: the way organs develop, how appetite signals get released in the brain, how genes are activated, even the metabolic chemistry inside a baby's cells. Research shows that the environment of the womb helps determine how a baby's metabolism is put together, or programs it for later health. The science of fetal programming is now widely accepted.

Doctors used to think of body fat as nothing more than inert insulation, but they know now that fat is an active tissue that releases hormones and plays a key role in keeping metabolism running. The amount of weight gain is critical. Women who gain too much weight are likely to have large babies. Weight gain should come slowly. Now here's where current diet takes over from genetic disposition. Normal weight women (BMI (body mass index) of 19.8 – 25) should gain no more than 25-35 pounds during pregnancy. Overweight women (BMI of 26-29) should gain no more than 15-25 pounds during pregnancy. Obese women (BMI greater than 29) should gain no more than 10-15 pounds during

Many women see pregnancy as a time they can eat anything, and that it will not affect the health of their babies. That has now been proven to be wrong. Obese women may pass along their obesity gene, but those genes will not be expressed (turned on) if the mother eats and exercises properly and gains minimal weight during pregnancy.

In a ground-breaking experiment, researchers began with pairs of fat yellow mice known as agouti mice. So called because they carry a particular gene - the agouti gene – making the rodents ravenous and prone to cancer and diabetes. Most of their offspring are identical to their parents. However, by feeding the mother mouse a diet rich in methyl donors (small chemical clusters that can attach to a gene and turn it off) starting just before conception the babies were born lean, with no predisposition toward cancer or diabetes. These methyl molecules are common in the environment and are found in many foods. Stay tuned for the release of my new book: "The Methyl Diet: turning off the hunger gene."

After being consumed by the mothers, the methyl donors worked their way into the developing embryos' chromosomes and onto the critical agouti gene. The mothers passed along the agouti gene to the children, but thanks to the methyl-rich pregnancy diet, they added to the gene a chemical switch that dimmed the gene's deleterious effects. A subtle nutritional change in the pregnant mother rat had a dramatic impact on the gene expression of the baby!

The science lies in the fact that while genes pass down traits, genes themselves need instructions for what to do, and where and when to do it. These instructions are found not in the letters of the DNA itself, but in an array of chemical markers know collectedly as the epigenome. The epigenic switches and markers help switch on or off the expression of particular genes.

Fact: the epigenome is just as critical as the DNA to the healthy development of organisms, human included. Epigenic signals can be passed on from one generation to the next, sometimes for several generations, without changing a single genes sequence. What is eye-opening is a growing body of evidence suggesting that the epigenic changes wrought by one's diet, behavior, and surrounding can echo far into the future. Put simply, what you eat today can affect the health and behavior of your great grandchildren.

The commonly held belief is that through our DNA we are destined to have a particular body shape, personate, and disease. Some scholars even contend that the genetic code predetermines intelligence and is the root cause of many social ills, including poverty, crime, and valence. Gene as fate had become conventional wisdom. But through the study of epigenic, that notion at last may be proved outdated.

Epigenetics introduces the concept of free will into our idea of genetics. People used to think that once your genetic code was laid down in early development that was it for life. To be clear: cancer is not genetic, it is epigenic. Common signaling pathways know to lead to cancerous tumors also activate DNA-methylation machinery; knocking out one of the enzymes in that pathway prevents the tumors from developing.

People can maintain the integrity of the epigenome through diet. Lifelong methylation diets may be the key to staying thin, healthy, and living a long life.

Further, recent studies have documented that women can influence the birth weight and metabolism of their babies with caffeine. Two to three small cups (100 mg.) of coffee a day will boost the metabolism of both mother and child, overcoming the effects of fluoridation and lack of exercise. Now, if obesity was genetic, then nothing you can do during your pregnancy would affect your child's health. While still controversial, these programs deserve serious consideration.

So what does get passed down?

What does occur is that the habits of parents get passed down to the children. That's right, habits. Parents mean well, but either they cannot control their own poor eating habits and pass that behavior on, or they want to show how much they love their children by indulging them, or they simply give up, unable to fight the constant messages and temptations offered by the media, malls, and mass marketers. It's pretty hard to fight off 15,000 messages a day when the average parent spends only 4 minutes a day talking to their children who rarely, if ever, hear educational or opposing view messages.

Further argument against genetic-based obesity

In 1950 there was far less obesity just a century ago. In the early 1900s only 1 in 150 people were obese. In the 1950s less than 10% of the population was classified as such. Genetic changes take tens or even hundreds of thousands of years to evolve, certainly not a hundred years. And these are just some of the many arguments that I have used to refute mainstream medicine and restore my patients' hope and faith.

Caffeine and the medical / scientific community

One reason that you may not have heard about the many benefits of caffeine is a lack of economic incentive. There is no real benefit for any company to conduct the required scientific studies. The studies themselves are quite costly and the companies are not compensated for doing such work. The benefits of caffeine, though profound, are not profitable. Further, any profit from a caffeine pill would be little.

It is also a long and costly venture to prove to the Food and Drug Administration (FDA) the benefits of a substance. Extensive scientific research and a mountain of paperwork are necessary to make any such suggestion to the FDA.

Caffeine is on the FDA safe list known as the substances that are "Generally Recognized as Safe" or the GRAS. It has been on the GRAS list for over two decades. The list allows for the ability of food and drink makers to put caffeine in their products because it is considered safe.

One regulation set by the FDA is that caffeine can be labeled as an alertness aid but all the other benefits we will be discussing throughout this book cannot be promoted as benefits of caffeine in any commercially labeled product.

That is the intention of this book: to give you the whole picture on caffeine. This is not simply my opinion but scientific facts that have been long known by both the medical and scientific community.

Even in the face of all the new data it is truly a wonder that people fear the effects of caffeine. Large numbers of the population limit the amount of coffee they drink each day or monitor how much caffeine is in other beverages they consume. They feel because of what they've been told that they should avoid caffeine because it is dangerous.

People often try to "quit" caffeine as if they are giving up a dangerous nicotine addiction. The reason for this is simply lack of information. This book is aimed at providing the necessary information so that people know and understand the many unspoken benefits that come from caffeine use and learn that they do not need to be afraid of caffeine.

It is not just the average man or woman who is misinformed. There are many in the medical profession, including physicians, that have outdated, unproven studies that they rely on. This misinformation, along with certain advocacy groups, puts forth a picture of caffeine to the public that would make anyone question the consequences of caffeine use.

Just enter the word into a search engine on the internet and your screen will be flooded with all types of data listing the dangers of caffeine use. You can find claims that it causes heart problems, hypertension, anxiety and dehydration. These are just a few of the common problems that are wrongly attributed to caffeine use.

We will be separating facts from fiction and discussing many popular myths about caffeine as well as coffee and other popular caffeinated beverages. Caffeine is one of the most misunderstood substances in our society despite its popularity around the world.

Why do we know so little about caffeine?

Caffeine has the ability to suppress the appetite and increase energy. Imagine if you will the impact of a drug as inexpensive as caffeine with this ability would have on drug companies with patents on high cost weight loss products. Then consider the impact of having a low-cost highly effective drug that suppresses the appetite would have on food companies. We have to face some cold hard facts; and the truth is food companies don't want people to eat less, and drug companies don't want any more competition than they already have.

Drug Companies

A true cure to obesity would threaten drug companies, the food industry, and even the government. This is a secret that they don't want people to figure out.

Drug companies have one goal, which is to keep people using on whatever drugs they can get them hooked on. They want people taking their pills on a long term, preferably life-long basis, because that means long term profit for them.

A cure to diseases, or the ability to prevent diseases all together, would mean one thing to drug companies: a huge profit loss and eventual bankruptcy. This would have an obvious negative impact on our economy and that would not be good for those in power.

Drug companies have a long history of lying about the effectiveness of their products. They lie even more when it comes to advertising the safety of them. It is the aim of those companies to make a drug appear better than it is, while comparing it to the negative effects of a drug put forth by a competitor. This of course is a natural part of the business world, but taken to an unnatural level in the drug industry.

The Food Industry

The food industry has long been known to purposely create foods that are addicting. They use products known to increase hunger, and whether it makes us fat or not is of little concern to them. They, like the drug companies, are interested in profit and do what they need to do to ensure that we as a nation stay fat.

Consider that the main goal is to have people buying more food. This is done by creating the addictive foods which increase hunger. When you consider the levels of additives in most foods today it is shocking. There are high levels of high-fructose corn syrup, artificial sweeteners, and thousands upon thousands of other man-made chemicals in much of the food we consume on a regular basis.

The effect these man-made chemicals have on the human body can be explained in simple terms: they make us fat. They affect the functioning of our thyroid and hypothalamus, making them operate improperly and creating obesity.

The Weight Loss / Money Gain Industry

Few people realize that most weight loss companies are owned and operated by either the food industry or the drug industry. This is one more dirty little secret they don't want people to know about. The weight loss industry cashes in on hundreds of billions of dollars each year from people desperate to lose weight. These profits go right back into the very industries that created the problem in the first place.

The weight loss industry has become one of largest markets in the world. U.S. corporations now see the promise of profit is huge in the global arena. The one requirement for them to continue making billions of dollars is that people continue to keep getting and staying fat.

Eliminate the Threat

When you consider the billions and billions of dollars at stake, it seems logical that these companies are willing to do whatever it takes to eliminate any threats. A scientific study or a company coming forth with a true cure for the weight issue has to be either discredited or eliminated.

We must also look at the effect a weight loss cure would have on the multi-billion dollar patent industry. Drug companies spend millions of dollars to obtain patents and promote the safety of surgical procedures. The FDA approves these patents and procedures. If a drug like caffeine came along with no patent and was proved to be a true weight loss cure then suddenly these companies have spent their millions and billions of dollars in vain. You would suddenly see less of these outrageous commercials suggesting that surgery alone is going to cure your weight problem; that is, of course, if it doesn't kill you first. The FDA approves these surgeries while at the same time warning you about the affects of caffeine.

So we see that if a cure to weight loss was found, drug companies lose billions. Sure mankind might be saved but that means little to these companies. They don't have to care because they are only obliged to focus on earnings. They are often owned or linked to other publicly traded corporations and this creates a situation where they just care about profits, not the effects their drugs are having on society.

One way of seeing how desensitized these companies are is to consider that they refer to mankind simply as "consumers". This is a word used by both the government and corporations. Consumers don't have feelings, consumers buy products. Consumers spend billions of dollars to keep corporations, and those invested in them, rich. Meanwhile people are needlessly dying of obesity.

It is also tragic that it is man-made products that are killing man. Man-made products cause clogged colons, ineffective thyroids, and hormonal imbalances just to name a few. It is the consumption of foods injected with thousands of man-made chemicals that cause so many of our worlds' health problems. Then we take prescription and nonprescription drugs that actually make things worse in the long run for us. We treat our dry skin with man-made lotions and creams that have chemicals that make us sick.

Then to treat our dehydration we consume water that is often treated with fluoride. The very fluoride that we put in our water to "treat" it is responsible for sluggishness, poor circulation, lack of oxygen in the blood and many other things that negatively affect weight loss. These are some of the other issues that we will discuss as we get further in the book. There is much more to be said about fluoride.

Separating the myths from the facts

Caffeine is far more than a "wake me up" substance. Its benefits are no less than amazing, life-changing, one of the most medicinal, beneficial substances ever provided by nature. This book will provide the scientific verification of the amazing properties of caffeine and tell us precisely how to use this little understood chemical, and we will debunk all the myth concerning this panacea.

The four great myths of caffeine are:

1) That it's bad for your heart
2) That it increase anxiety
3) That it causes dehydration
4) That it negatively affects blood pressure

But before we debunk those myths and detail the proper methodology for taking and monitoring the use of caffeine, let's review the history of coffee and caffeine. Take the time to read the book. However, if you're desperate to begin today, then go to chapter fifteen and start there. For those with more patience, you will find the material presented to be fascinating and educational.

CHAPTER ONE

From Cave Man To Café

I believe humans get a lot done, not because we're smart, but because we have thumbs so we can make coffee. ~Flash Rosenberg

Caffeine dates back as early as 700,000 B.C. There are campsite remnants that make it realistic for anthropologists to believe that Stone Age man may have chewed the seeds, roots, bark, and leaves of many plants and maybe even ground up the caffeine-bearing plant material into a paste before ingestion.

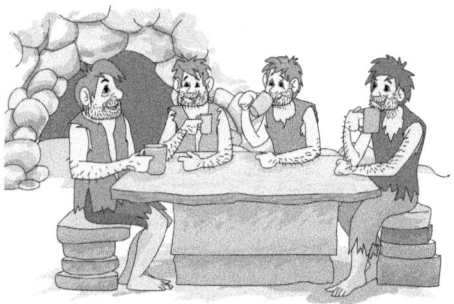

Evidence suggests the modern day brewing process may have gotten its beginnings with the technique of infusing plant material with hot water, which used higher temperatures to extract the caffeine. This technique was discovered many years later but eventually gave birth to the most popular and familiar caffeine-containing beverages, coffee, tea, chocolate, cola, and many others.

This book is aimed at telling the whole story concerning the history, uses, dangers, and benefits of caffeine. While fully considering the health effects of caffeine, we will take a closer look at this drug that has captivated men and women in every strata of society for thousands of years.

Nearly 90% of Americans use caffeine daily. However few people really know much about caffeine despite its rank as the world's most popular and most used drug. Caffeine is a vegetable alkaloid crystallizing in white silky needle, found in the leaves and seeds of the coffee and tea plants.

Caffeine has overcome other addictive psychoactive substances in the fact that it is accessible almost anywhere in the world with no regulations, readily available to adults and children. In fact the most popular drinks in the world: coffee, tea, and cola all contain significant amounts of caffeine.

With its popularity and acceptance today it is hard to believe that once upon a time coffee was placed in the same category as drugs like LSD. The controversy over caffeine can be found dating back to the 1600s in England where on one hand people were warned that it was a health hazard linked to depression, and on the other they were told it was an antidote to the bubonic plague.

Introducing the World's Most Popular Drink

Europe was introduced to coffee and tea during the seventeenth century and to this day it has become a cornerstone of European culture. In English an Arabian medical text it was reported that coffee caused headaches, insomnia and feelings of discontent. These reports were spread from the introduction of the drink. In contrast to these reports, during the 1600s coffee was recommended in fighting against the bubonic plague, which at the time was in the process of killing a quarter of Europe's population. In the western world, consumption of coffee and tea has become such a part of life that in the twenty-first century it is the biggest cash crop on planet earth, and tea is the world's most popular drink.

Coffee and tea have always been recognized as drugs. Coffee, not unlike other drugs, is an intoxicant. It is used as a euphoric social and physical stimulant, as well as a digestive aid. In their early years coffee, tea, and cola elixirs were used almost exclusively as medicines. Scientists have now isolated the pharmacologically active constituent. The health claims for tea are even older than those of coffee. A Chinese dictionary, describes preparing an elixir by boiling raw, green tea leaves in kettles.

Reports from the early 19th century state that caffeine was first isolated in coffee, and at that time scientists began to study the drug. It is classified as a central nervous system stimulant with the ability to restore strength and vigor. Pure caffeine is highly toxic and bitter; once ingested it is absorbed and distributed quickly into the bloodstream.

Caffeine: a lethal drug?

There is no question that caffeine is a potent and potentially lethal drug. The lethal dose for a healthy adult male is estimated at less than 15 grams. When you consider that about five cups of coffee can cause severe reactions - like insomnia, ear ringing, diarrhea, even irregular heartbeat - you realize the potential of caffeine when consumed in unrealistic quantities. Hemorrhaging and convulsing can occur in cases of extreme intoxification. Another sign of caffeine's obvious status as a drug is the withdrawal symptoms that users experience when they stop using caffeine. Symptoms such as headaches, irritability, and difficulty concentrating are commonly found when people stop drinking coffee. This is one of many reasons that on our program we will be recommending using only trace doses of caffeine; far less than any level of concern, so there is little danger of any side effects.

Health Benefits Linked to Caffeine

What about the health benefits of caffeine which are rarely talked about? Medical studies in the 20th century conclude there is much evidence linking caffeine to lowering rates of suicide and cirrhosis of the liver. It has also been credited with creating more efficient use of glycogen and blood sugars. There are even reports that it can improve short-term memory, enhance ones athletic abilities, even alleviate asthmatic symptoms. Many other such claims about the benefits of caffeine use can be found throughout history. These findings will be supported or debunked later in the book.

The Original Starbucks

During the 1600s coffee and tea were introduced to Europe by Dutch traders. In the mid-1600s a London pub owner was rumored to be among the first to serve tea. Among the many reasons for its popularity were claims from as early as 2737 B.C. that tea quenched thirst and lessened the desire for sleep. Other reports from the 1600s suggested the use of tea and coffee as a remedy for acidity. One report suggests they were used as blood purifiers as well. In Europe, despite its high cost, the use of tea spread quickly throughout all levels of society and along with coffee becoming one of Europe's favorite beverages.

Bohemianism was entering English society, especially its universities in the middle 1600s. During the same time period the first English coffeehouse was opened in Oxford and shortly after came the first London coffeehouse. Over the next fifty years an exciting and new chapter in literary and social history took place as these English coffee-houses served coffee, tea and chocolate, becoming places where people of all ages and all walks of life began to socially interact. These interactions would be at the root of the popularity and the controversy of the coffeehouse.

The First Chocolate Addicts

It was neither coffee nor tea though that introduced caffeine into European bloodstreams; chocolate was introduced more than fifty years earlier. Who could resist the chocolate coming from South America by the Spaniards, which was often served in distinguished coffeehouses like London's Cocoa Tree, a popular hangout for the literary giants of the eighteenth century? You may wonder, with its much lower dose of caffeine, why chocolate became so popular. Its reputation is much accredited to its ability, thru theobromine, to enhance and accelerate the effects of caffeine. This made it rival the popularity of other beverages with much higher caffeine content.

Was there life before caffeine?

Today, in every American city, caffeine is used readily on a daily basis by large masses of the population. The ancient Turkish coffeehouse tradition of meeting to dish the dirt and catch up what was going on in politics around the world is now a way of life in American society. Workplaces everywhere in the western world have break rooms with coffee makers, tea pots, and chocolate in one form or another.

The Cloud of Mystery

A European chemist in 1819 was the first to name and isolate caffeine. The young physician, Friedlieb Runge, discovered that caffeine had the ability to alter ones mood and stimulate its users. He found these attributes in both coffee and tea. Caffeine was isolated from cola nuts and mate, a plant used to make an energizing beverage. There was a report in London's Daily News about caffeine, and it seemed the world was long awaiting its discovery.

There is much mystery surrounding the origins of coffee, tea, and chocolate. We know without a doubt that the three plants were being used long before anyone in Europe even heard of them. From natives of Arabia to savages in early America the many effects of these plants were long recognized. There are European and Arab scholars that believe lost African documents surely would prove that coffee was well known long before the 15th century. However there is little hard proof to support this. So until now you may have never have known - as you read your morning paper and enjoy your cup of tea or coffee - there was a great mystery surrounding their epic journey to America. It wasn't until around 1450 that documents show any knowledge of the coffee tree in Greek, Roman, African, or Middle Eastern worlds. Even though we know coffee was indigenous in the Arab world, and that it grows throughout the Middle East and all over the mountains of the Africa, there is no substantial physical evidence to support its use before that time.

The Dancing Goat

There are many stories about how the first cup of coffee came into the world. Here we will explore some of the strangest and most popular myths. One suggests that a holy man had a cat who he trained to carry the seeds of the coffee plant to mountains in Ethiopia. The story goes that this cat journeyed all over central Africa and into the remote mountain regions of Ethiopia. It was there that the plant was cultivated and later purchased by an Arab merchant who brought the plant back to Arabia. It was then soon thereafter that the plant was introduced to the rest of the world.

Who can resist the myth of the Ethiopian goat herder and his strange dancing goats? It is a story often found in Western literature. The tale relates that the goat herder noticed his herd eating berries and then acting hyper, even dancing around.

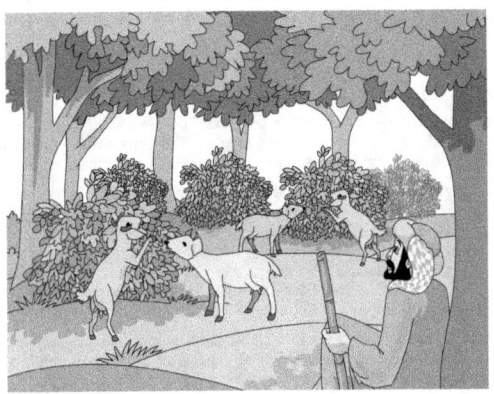

Curious about the behavior of his dancing goats, he naturally decided to try it for himself. However when he told his story to a nearby holy man, the holy man threw his "evil" berries into the fire. When the enticing aroma filled the room the goat herder saw more potential in the beans. He took what was left of his catch and dissolved them in hot water and the result: the world's first cup of coffee. This story is a well known and believed account of how coffee was discovered. Both tales make one believe that it was indeed the remote Ethiopians who were the first to have recognized the powerful effects of the coffee plant.

The Coffee Cats

The facts that the beans are said to have a skin covering proved to be very important. In the 18th century, coffee seedlings were first introduced in certain tropical countries. Some link the proliferation of the plant in these parts to the eating habits of the native feline. Like the African feline, these cats enjoyed the fruit and spread the seeds in its excrement. There are only three known species of the civet cat in the genus, and the one reported to have spread the seeds was in the Viverridae family. It is a relative of the mongooses, civets, and genets. Two of the species are known only in the West Indies, and the other is found throughout the Middle East. It is also known as a musang or toddy cat.

The animal is not really a cat. It has catlike features including its face and long colored fur. It has stripes and spots as well as a long tail. These animals live to be between four to ten years of age and grow up to two and half feet long while weighing only six to seven pounds. They feed on smaller animals but also eat vegetation, which is how the rumors of their vital role in the history of caffeine came about.

Other Animals and the History of Coffee

There are other animals, including monkeys and birds that are known for eating the coffee berry. These animals also play a role in the history of coffee. They are not able to digest the beans and so they are passed through in the excrement. They are gathered and then recycled and turned into a coffee referred to as "monkey coffee". A 20th century writer refers to the relationship between coffee and animals. He claims that birds and cats are said to have spread coffee throughout many lands.

Coffee a Weapon

There are stories that Ethiopian soldiers then and now who have used the berries to form small balls used during battle to help fight thirst and fatigue. The balls were formed by mixing the seeds along with animal lard and then grinding the two ingredients with stone into tiny balls.

Soldiers in Africa traveling through barren deserts took nothing to eat except the coffee balls, and they claimed that only one ball could support them for a whole day. It also improved mood, which helped to fight the terrible conditions they faced. Having to choose what little would be taken with them, it speaks volumes that they chose to carry the coffee balls rather than meat. When you consider this choice you must believe that the effects were obviously dramatic. These soldiers believed strongly enough in them that they risked their lives by depending on the tiny balls to provide enough substance for survival.

We can guess from coffee's emergence throughout Africa that it was growing and being cultivated. But despite all the legends, there is no direct evidence that shows coffee's roots in Africa any earlier than the seventeenth century. Even though we can estimate that as far back as the creation of the Pyramids, through the rise and fall of the Roman Empire, and during the start of the Middle Ages, coffee was most likely being enjoyed in one form or another.

So why the delay?

It was hundreds of years from the Ethiopians to the entry of coffee into the rest of the world, even though Ethiopia was known to the rest of the Middle East for at least three thousand years. We would expect that even with the African continent being so vast and dangerous for travel, they would have been aware of coffee.

Despite the likelihood that most natives had limited contact with one another, they must have had many interactions with European and Middle-Eastern traders. And so the traders must have had knowledge of the Ethiopian tribes. But if we rely only on what can be documented, there was no knowledge of coffee among the Europeans or Middle Easterners of the time.

To Tea or Not to Tea

One of the oldest documents that speaks of coffee is titled *The Canon of Medicine,* written sometime in the late 9th century. It refers to the term "buncham," stating that "buncham" was good for the stomach and it was a hot and dry beverage. There is some speculation about the meaning of the Arabic words "bunn" and "buncham," but it is believed by many scholars that they refer to the coffee berry and to coffee the beverage. The journal refers to almost 800 different drugs, and there are more than just a few mentions of the term "buncham."

The journal refers to almost 800 different drugs, and there are more than just a few mentions of the term "buncham."

In two separate chapters there is an entry for *buncham,* speaking to the medicinal properties of both *bunn* and *buncham.* The first description in Europe came from a German physician who saw the beverage prepared in Aleppo in the later 1500s. The first description in Europe came believed by many scholars that they refer to the coffee berry and to coffee the beverage.

He wrote also that in this same water they take a fruit called *Bunn.* We can assume he was acquainted with the *Canon of Medicine* because, upon its translation, it had become a well respected medical journal in Europe and around the world. It was required in many medical schools to read the Canon at that time until the 17th century.

Doctors were also encouraged to read a journal titled *Wholesome Advise against the Abuse of Hot Liquors, Particularly of Coffee, Chocolate, Tea.* And it was often a part of medical students' suggested reading until the mid 1600s

The Religious World Welcomes Caffeine

With all these mentions of caffeine and coffee, the greater mystery surrounds the lack of any records in the Middle East and Europe. Eventually caffeine would become of great intrigue to the Islamic world, where the use of alcohol was strictly forbidden.

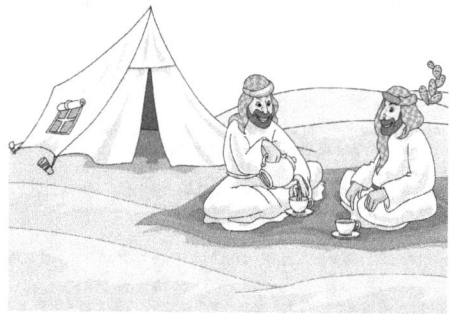

Christians in Europe also eagerly embraced coffee's arrival for many of the same reasons. At that time water was feared due to contamination and spread of disease, and beer was the primary drink, for that was consumed at most meals.

One must consider the pleasure that coffee must have provided in these circles where the rules were so strict about what was perceived as permissible and what was strictly forbidden. The arrival of a beverage that not only tasted good, but had the ability to alter ones mood, was welcomed with open arms among both religious societies.

After being so well received by the Islamic and Christian circles one would believe that it was just a matter of time before the drink would spread throughout society.

However, for reasons unknown, it would be more than 500 years before coffee would gain in popularity and become commonplace in the Arabian and European world. Yet another mystery is that apparently the Arabs knew about Chinese tea. In fact there are reports dating to around 800 A.D that state taxes from tea levies were an important source of revenue. We believe from the findings a quote that they were familiar with the effects of tea. Consider a line from the late 1400's which states "The people of China are accustomed to use as a beverage an infusion of a plant, which they call *sakh*."

With this revelation it becomes clear that they knew of the drink and the effects of it. This being so, it becomes even more suspicious that they didn't know about coffee. The reason for the mystery is due to the fact that tea was another world away. Not just a world away, but located in a land where few had ever traveled. Few interactions with the Chinese are known to have occurred at that time.

They were aware of tea, which we know to have been growing in a nearby region, and they were familiar with people whom they interacted with on regular occasions, but coffee remained unknown to them. The mystery remains as to why the Arabs seemingly knew nothing of coffee when it seems so logical that they should have.

Coffee: The Gods and the Bible

Possibly to avoid the embarrassment that the lack of knowledge pertaining to coffee created, there are those who would suggest its mention in ancient Hebrew and Greek chronicles. These references seem to agree on one point, which is coffee's ability to alter the mood of its users and of its definition as a drug.

With the obsession over what was permissible according to religious teachings and what was not, we would expect that if coffee was mentioned in books such as the Koran and the Bible, we would be well aware of it. Yet the myths are abundant.

Some would even suggest that in the epic the Odyssey, the drink served by Helen referred to as nepenthe was actually a mixture of both wine and coffee. The references to its ability to alter the mood of any who drank it makes one believe that it was a much stronger combination of drugs than mere coffee and wine.

We can assume that perhaps coffee was one of many ingredients in drinks that included other drugs such as heroin or cocaine. One would not relate coffee with the ability to cure pain or eliminate worry, which is the meaning of "nepenthes," so again there had to be a stronger combination at work. We learn from Homer that nepenthe was used in Egypt and Ethiopia, and again the rumors that he is referring to coffee can be argued with the description of the drink's ability to alter mood. References to the drink's ability to make a person incapable of shedding any tears, even if a loved one died before their eyes, again suggests coffee.

Coffee: the Drug, the Drink, the Myth

From the 1600s to the 1700s in Europe there were several theories about the drugs of that time, and one Swiss writer credited coffee as a stimulant, while at the same time cautioning users that it was a dangerous drug and that its benefits had been greatly exaggerated.

There were claims of noblemen drinking coffee leading back to Greece. And what many believed to be another exaggerated tale told of a famous Sultan who insisted on having drunk coffee all over the Near East, saying it was famed among the Spartans. Some scholars even went as far as to claim that there were stories of coffee drinking in the Old Testament, stating David used it as a gift to settle an argument with one of his enemies.

Another Middle Eastern story in Islam tells of the archangel Gabriel using coffee to cure illness, going from town to town hailing the drink as a cure all. It was even suggested that the archangel brought the drink to earth to save Mohammed who was suffering from self diagnosed narcolepsy, but apparently was cured by just a sip of hot coffee. There is yet another myth that Mohammed was to have felt such energizing vigor from the drink, that once, near death, he could drink coffee and take on any feat with his new found strength.

There may be some truth to the tale of a holy man and healer being the first Arab to discover the wild berries. When he threw them into the fire and drank the mixture that remained, the story began. He shared this drink with his fellows who liked the drink so much that over time he gained much notoriety that eventually a place of worship was built in his name. This can be documented with enough prevalence that there may be more fact than fiction in the legend.

The First Coffeehouse

During the 1500s, a Sufi whom had fallen ill after traveling in Ethiopia recalled that while staying there he had been given a beverage known as "qahwa." In his recollection this beverage made him feel energized and light in spirit. He drank of it and again felt the effects so much so that he was no longer ill. He shared this story and the drink with his fellows, and this gave way to the Sufi people falling in love with coffee. It became a regular part of the all night prayer sessions, and the stories of the drink's benefits quickly spread throughout the land.

Prayer was an integral part of their society, and the long hours of prayer required energy and concentration. Whether this made coffee a Godsend or not is up for discussion. In any case this gave way to the first coffeehouses being built. Soon, all over the Islamic world, everyone was drinking coffee.

However, some orthodox Muslims said that according to the Koran coffee should be banned because of its ability to alter ones mood. They looked at it the same as other drugs like alcohol and opiates and feared the effects its use would have upon the culture.

Coffee Gaining Approval

In the 1600s doctors and religious men in the capital cities of the holy land gave their approval of coffee. This gave way to the coffeehouse being introduced in Constantinople. Prominent business leaders of the time started cashing in on the popularity of the drink and the places where it was being consumed. Some leaders of the Sufi sect strongly encouraged the use of caffeine and promoted its effects, but again caffeine met opposition by other religious leaders. Despite the best efforts of some Islamic leader, in just a few hundred years the Islamic world was filled with coffee-houses, and in Constantinople alone there were hundreds of them.

Egypt Cashes In

All over the region began opening coffeehouses in all cities and towns, large and small. The Turks often assembled at the coffeehouses and they were especially popular among travelers. In Egypt, and other surrounding cities, coffee booths even offered delivery and take out services in the upper class areas. It was rumored that those who couldn't afford the beverage on a regular basis did whatever they could to buy just a single cup.

In Egypt, and throughout the region, coffee was actually sold from houses as well as tiny stalls and shops. Coffee was becoming quite popular among the upper class. This tradition has continued through modern times, and to this day coffee is still being sold the same way on almost every continent.

The Great Debate Continues

The debate over its benefit and safety didn't die with the birth of the coffeehouse. If anything it added fuel to the fire from which one side argued coffee was a god-given drink not forbidden by any religious scriptures, and the other side that argued the altering ones mood was certain to lead to sin. A head of the religious community said in a lesson that society was becoming filled with violence and noise due to the use of coffee, and he encouraged his parish not to partake.

One man attempting to create peace among the two opposing sides of the issue invited those most opposed to the use of coffee to his home. He served the beverage to them all. After drinking it himself, he refrained from any argument with them about its dangers. This left the men virtually speechless and his actions truly spoke louder than any of the words others who were speaking against coffee. The result of this important meeting was that coffee was no longer frowned upon and it seemed to resolve the conflict between the two opposing sides...at least for that moment.

This peace was short lived though as the popularity of coffee spread like wild fire. There were reports that people were spending all their time in coffeehouses consuming the beverage and held no reverence for the Sabbath. This became cause for concern. Another possible reason for the reemergence of the religious society frowning upon its use was that in Cairo not having the proper stash of coffee became legal grounds for ending ones marriage.

According to his teachings, Mohammed had forbidden the use of any carbonized substance and this along with the lack of any mention of coffee in the Koran became a new basis for even stricter laws prohibiting the use of coffee and of coffeehouses.

Many believed that one reason for this new focus on coffee as such a sinful beverage had more to do with a certain leader of the time who was rumored to have murdered his entire family to take the throne. Attempting to divert attention from himself by blaming coffee, he spread fear about consequences users would face. His extreme measures seemed to work at deterring coffee drinking in the open.

Behind Closed Doors

Coffee drinking, of course, continued behind closed doors and little was done by law enforcement of the time to abolish its use, although both coffee and coffeehouses were strictly banned towards the end of the 16th century by this same leader. It was his fear that his own scandalous past was being discussed in coffeehouses, and so he ordered that they be shut down. The main result was that people just began to drink their coffee at home. One can look at the prohibition efforts with alcohol and see a common thread with the cause and effect of attempts at prohibiting the use of caffeine.

A Capital Offense

In the mid 17th century coffee, tobacco, and many other substances became the subject of another strict ban, and this time it became a capital offense to use them. The ban served as a major deterrent. Spies were sent to coffeehouses to see what was being discussed and there were religious men sent to try to change any topic away from politics. This lessened the occurrence of any noticeable social upheaval that was so feared by leaders of the time.

In the Islamic world, even those who had once so warmly embraced coffee had become fearful that the gatherings in the coffeehouses would lead to social unrest. The custom of the time was for people to lead fairly private lives, only entertaining a few guests at ones home for special occasions. The sudden, drastic change that came with the large gatherings at coffeehouses, along with the strict bans and fear the government was spreading, served to create much skepticism among the Islamic world in regards to coffee and the coffeehouse.

Eventually coffee was accepted as a drug of the purest form by the same people who once said it wasn't mentioned in the Koran. They now said that not only was it mentioned, but that in the afterlife there would be a coffeehouse in heaven. The popularity of the coffeehouse, and its use as a place for people to meet socially and discuss the news of the day, again was renewed, and the influence of this can be seen today around the world.

Throughout time, the place where writers, poets, doctors, lawyers, and every day workers came to meet was no longer the local pub but the coffeehouse. One could come not just to enjoy their favorite beverage or to catch up on the latest goings on in the political world, but to relax and listen to music or poetry.

We don't have to look far to see how this has influenced our culture today. Take a step into your local coffeehouse and you are sure to either hear music and poetry or find postings community events. The artistic crowd along with the white collar worker sitting at his table with his laptop computer and internet connection are as common in today's coffeehouse as the coffee itself.

A 21st Century Ban on Caffeine?

Without having faced the more dramatic bans of caffeine during our time we may easily scoff at the earlier challenges faced by the coffee drinkers. But even to this day, depending on the popular view of the time, those in power either praise coffee and caffeine, or look to it as cause for concern and attempt to moderate its use. This occurs all over the world.

27

There are even groups much like Alcoholics Anonymous but for coffee users, and with the use of the web people seek to make others "aware of the danger" of caffeine use, as if they were discussing heroin addiction. In a society that has become prevalent with banning the use of any substance that is deemed harmful, we must realize that it is not that farfetched to believe that one day coffee could again be on the long list of banned substances. One thing we now about history is its tendency to repeat itself.

A Travelers Account

The reports that came from European travelers who instinctively were curious about the traditions practiced in other cultures were vast and detailed. They reported that Islamic towns showed two extreme class differences in their coffeehouses.

You were either drinking coffee in back alley warehouses with lower class men of questionable merit - along with other travelers quite content to just sit around and indulge in the beverage and do little if nothing else - or you had to go to the other extreme and visit the more swanky end of town and dare you not to offer to buy the next round of coffee if you saw someone you knew in the ritzy establishment.

You had to have the money to uphold the image one was attempting to create by being seen in these high-end coffeehouses. There are many documented tales of these Islamic coffeehouses that came from the Europeans all telling, in one way or another, about the class differentiation in the establishments at that time. These differences continue to this day.

The Many Uses of the Coffee Berry

Arab traders discovered that by drying the husk of the coffee berry they could make a tea-like drink that they named "kisher," which was a tea-like beverage. The process used to create the drink consisted of boiling unripe coffee beans. There was even a wine made in parts of Africa around 900 A.D. using the fermented coffee berry. Still another drink, which they named "bounya," might be compared to drinking coffee grounds was created. These drinks were actually quite popular for many years until the process of infusion for making coffee was discovered many years later in the 1700s.

Mystery Around Tea

There is as much mystery surrounding just how and when tea was introduced to China as there is in why it took so long for the discovery of coffee in the West. Many believe that the Chinese were introduced to tea either from the tribesmen in India or Asia. Tales of the tribesmen boiling tea leaves over fire are found throughout Chinese literature. Some stories relate that it was monks who are due the credit. Much like the myths about coffee, we have no real proof to tell us just exactly how and when tea was introduced into Chinese culture, although it is much newer than one might think.

In its beginnings, tea, like coffee, was used only for its medical properties, such as its ability to help with digestion and settle the nerves. It was also used to alleviate pain. One report suggests that a priest recommended to an emperor suffering from severe headaches to use tea; and as the story spread, the demand for tea was so great that the beginning of it being cultivated had arrived.

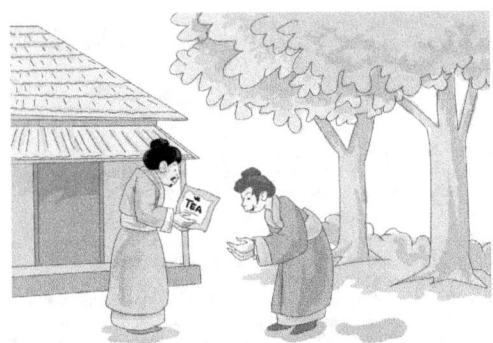

T'ang "Dynasty-Tea"

Tea was no question a remarkable and powerful ingredient in Chinese medicine; long before the T'ang dynasty. Tea was known to have many benefits, among those the ability to help with indigestion, weight loss, and fight diseases of the lungs as well as lower fever, and even as a treatment for epilepsy. This can be accounted for in ancient Chinese medical books. Our recent "revelations" of caffeine's ability to help burn fat and fight off the effects of smoking and lung disease are much less impressive in the light of the fact that this information has been around for at least 500 years.

Despite all this, legends still agree that the T'ang dynasty is responsible for the extreme popularity of tea in China today. Tea had a power and influence beyond measure. At that time, the T'ang dynasty was the richest in the world and the Japanese, wanting to imitate followed suit, began a love affair with tea as well. During the 1600s the birth and development of the teahouse, teagarden, and tea ceremony came to Japan.

Plotting a Revolution

The Russians followed suit, importing Chinese brick tea by the tons. This form of tea was made by drying the leaves and pressing them into a mold over fire, then placing the remains into baskets. They were then sold throughout the land. Tea was also consumed in cake form that people simply chewed. Other ingredients were added for flavor, including ginger, orange peel and many different spices. Eventually though the brick tea became less popular as powdered tea took over.

During the 1200s, Chinese teahouses, much like the coffeehouses in Islamic society, were opened. They also became places where people met to discuss politics and partake in social interactions on all levels. The records show that it was in a teahouse where the revolution of 1911 was plotted. Perhaps all that paranoia the early Islamics held had some relativity after all!

No one was traveling to China at that time, and it would be at least two thousand years after the Chinese discovered tea that anyone in Europe would know anything about it. The Arabs knew of tea hundreds of years before the Europeans. It is believed that they learned about tea in the

10th century. In the West, the first written document of tea came shortly before the Russians discovered it in the 16th century. Near the end of Ming's dynasty the first tea came from Amsterdam and was made from tea leaves imported from the Dutch.

Cacao in Mexico

Cacao has become very popular in Mexico. It is a drink given as charity to the poor. The cacao nuts are even used as currency. Only in recent times has the knowledge that it was in Mexican lowlands that cacao was first discovered and harvested into a chocolate drink come to light.

The Olmecs were the first to discover the cacao pods on the coasts of Mexico somewhere around 400 B.C., well before the Mayas arrival there. Before this discovery many thought that it was the Arabs or Chinese who were responsible for the discovery. cacao. It was quickly outlawed due to its ability to stimulate its users. Ironically, while banning its use for the rest of the land, the royals hoarded and used themselves. Eventually the royals made an exception for military persons to use and trade cacao beans in the hopes of establishing a good reputation among the other nations.

Chocolate and the Aztecs

In early Spanish reports it is rumored that many nobles had an addiction to chocolate. These reports suggest that some royalty began the day with large quantities of chocolate. They stated that much like common men would indulge in alcohol and other drugs when entertaining concubines, chocolate became a part of this routine. The addition of chocolate into these rituals may be attributed to its much known powers as an aphrodisiac.

Yet it was still only the royals and the military men that were enjoying the coca at this time. Remember that they knew nothing of the effects caffeine and theobromine had on the users. They believed that chocolate's effects were more mystical in nature and it was greatly valued as a drug.

One infamous report called chocolate the "drink of the gods," and at this time Cortes called the secret of chocolate's magical powers "theobroma cacao" (what became theobromine in modern times). A number of famous men of the time, including King Charles, Cortes, and King Ferdinand, were said to have been consumers of chocolate.

Columbus Discovers Chocolate

Most believe that it was the cacao seed that introduced caffeine into the life of Europeans. Along with the credit of finding America, it is Columbus who is said to have brought back the cacao bean in the 16th century during one of his many voyages.

Columbus returned to Spain with the cocoa pods and introduced the European world to its first taste of caffeine. It is unknown exactly who Columbus delivered the pods to, but what is clear is that by the mid 1500s the Spaniards had their first taste of chocolate. Soon, visiting westerners would be the first to introduce the cacao beans to Seville.

It is not certain that the Spanish understood the powers of the drink. Some called its use crazy and thought it was of no value. There were others simply disgusted with the chocolate, but over time both men and women would become addicted. They especially loved black chocolate. It was off the Honduran coast, in a Mayan trade, where Columbus is rumored to have discovered the cacao beans.

Chocolate Across the Atlantic

By the later part of the 17th century, men and women in Italy had become well acquainted with chocolate. Being only the second European country at the time to be aware of it, the fear of the unknown again became cause for religious concern. The concern was also due to the widespread use and popularity the chocolate had found among the people. Religious leaders were called to determine whether chocolate would be allowed during Lent, since it was considered a pleasurable experience in a time of chaste.

Poison

In Europe, sugar cane was available at a high price. It was being imported from the east and another mixture became the rage; it was a mix of cacao and sugar. Many used the cacao and added it to several other ingredients to create a variety of beverages. Chocolate was mainly enjoyed at room temperature or chilled at this time. For reasons unknown they hadn't really experimented with serving it hot. Once they began serving it hot, the popularity of the drink was even more dramatic.

In contrast to the way chocolate drinks are created today, in ancient times they were much more potent. The Europeans were aware of components beyond caffeine, what Cortes called theobromine. They found ways of preparing the beverage so that it packed a serious punch. The effect was often deadly as legend tells us. People used chocolate drinks to poison people because of its strong aroma and taste. It was the perfect combination to hide the poison. This was taking place for many years in Europe and tales relating this can be found throughout European literature

The Earliest Carb Counters

You may be surprised to learn that in the beginning chocolate was used to help during fasting. Now that's a diet anyone could handle. The paste created in making chocolate with various ingredients contained large amounts of carbohydrates, protein, and minerals. Naturally being a great help with fasting, it became popular among the religions that practiced and encouraged fasting. Chocolate still wasn't as popular among the upper class yet, but artists' portrayals of the time often contain the beverage being served along with breakfast.

In the 1500s chocolate remained relatively unknown outside of the Spanish culture. But as we may expect, you can't keep a secret that good for long. We know that in the 1600s Spain was a very popular place for the upper class and trendy people of the world to come and find the latest and greatest comestible. As it turned out, drinking hot chocolate was in, and so all those visiting Spain at this time were sure to take home with them some of the delicacy. And the notion that drinking it was a way to fit in among the rich and famous evolved. Also, because of the benefit chocolate gave in fasting, it was highly acclaimed in the Catholic community and among other religions, and has stood the test of time.

In the 1500s France was introduced to chocolate by Spanish religious men and, much like it had in Europe, it was only the upper class that really got to indulge.

It wasn't until around 1620 that chocolate filtered down to the masses in England, though there are reports it had been introduced many years earlier and that it was there by the mid 1500s. Why it took so long in England for chocolate to become popular we are unsure. However, unlike Spain and France, where only the rich and privileged of society could enjoy chocolate, in England it was available to everyone.

Chocolate was sold and served in stores there and the cost was affordable enough so that most everyone could at least try it once. Documents show the cost of chocolate in England at that time was around fifteen shillings a pound which was still fairly expensive but less expensive than it was in France and the rest of Europe.

In the middle of the 17th century, within just a few years of England opening its first coffeehouses, chocolate drinking became almost as popular as coffee. The popularity of chocolate as a beverage though didn't stand the test of time, and near the middle of the 18th century it was much less common.

A book written by Marco Polo documents his travels in Italy. He talks about all the trade of commerce taking place there. He mentions an imperial tax, but fails to make any mention of tea. No one is sure why Polo left tea out of his notes, but other writers in the 16th century made mention of the drink in the West. However not until the 17th century is there any mention of tea in East Indian Trading Company logs, yet know it was there and available to the upper class. We know it had a brief popularity in Paris in the 17th century as well. By the 18th century, tea had become the most popular drink in England, and created the most revenue from import.

The Coffee Break

Coffee may have had a great deal of competition, but its popularity dramatically increased among all classes in the 18th century. One writer stated that it had become so systemic that without it people just couldn't function. This same writer went on to complain about how workers had the tendency to take a break mid-morning to enjoy their coffee.

The Caffeine Blessing

There were many in the catholic world that felt caffeine was evil. The same old arguments that had taken place in Islamic nations began to occur in Europe until, during the middle of the 16th century, the Pope gave his blessing to caffeine. When the time came for the Pope to try the beverage for himself it is said that he found the drink so delightful he thought it would be more of a sin to not allow his fellow man to enjoy its splendor. He made the declaration that he found no reason for Christians to stay away from the drink.

Although many religious leaders had tried and failed at discouraging the use of caffeine, it seemed this Pope's blessing made a lasting impact. Keep in mind that prior to his blessing the revenue in coffee trade was at a minimum and it was still looked upon with great paranoia and distaste by many other religious leaders.

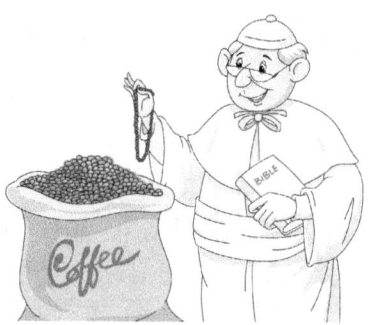

Many feel that because of his blessing the Pope spared Europe from many years of debate among the religious leaders that had occurred in Islamic nations. The Pope's edicts also spared Europe from all the bans and civic unrest that other nations had faced in the great debate over caffeine.

Near the end of the 17th century the first coffeehouse can be documented in Italy. We would imagine that, along with drinks like lemonade and tea, coffee was now being served.

The French Cafe

During the 18th century there were hundreds of cafes being opened in Paris and thousands by the 19th century. They had become even more popular than the coffee-houses of other countries. Many were erected to cater to the upper class and to the government leaders. Cafes had themes much like they do today in the western world. These cafes became places for the literary giants of the time to come and read their works. Great artists, both literary and canvas, lingered to discuss politics and enjoy the notoriety that went along with being associated with cafes that catered to famous people. Men like Victor Hugo, Napoleon, and many others including dukes and other nobles were regular attendees. One writer wrote that Paris had become one large café.

German Influence

It was a German housewife who changed everything with her invention of the filter drip coffee. There had been many others before her that had come close, all with the same idea, but it was this woman, Frau Melitta, who, in an effort to impress her husband, figured out how to do what no one before her had. She used blotting paper along with a pot that had a special bottom, and this combination worked to brew the first truly decent pot of coffee. Prior to this time the grounds always came through and so the coffee was usually quite bitter. When you truly imagine what a properly brewed cup of coffee tastes like compared to what had been, there is no comparison.

During this time people became known for what they loved. There was a certain sense of pride taken in advocating chocolate for instance. One man rose to royalty all by creating a chocolate revolution. Yet another man became famous for his love of coffee. These men, of course, often frequented the cafes of France and enjoyed life among the other rich and privileged. One café was the Café Florian which became famous in the 18th century. Anyone who was important in the world of literature or royalty visited this café. Artists and writers of all kinds flocked like a cult to this one establishment. It was like Berkeley in California: anybody who was anyone wanted to be seen there. There were many other famous cafes such as the Café Greco, but Café Florian was the most famous.

Drink Until You Can Drink No More

A physician of the 17th century advised not only his patients but the entire country to drink tea in excess. He suggested that a person should drink at least ten cups a day and then gradually increase that amount until you drank as much as your stomach could contain. This is documented in a medical journal and was actually advised.

From 1600s to 1700s the medical field was constantly debating the benefits and dangers of coffee, tea, and chocolate. They recognized the effects but not the properties responsible, and thus considered all three to be drugs to be prescribed by doctors and chemists. As all three became available to the public they also became popular in the Western world. Yet the debate continued as to whether caffeine was more harmful than helpful to the human body. Some claims

33

suggested that coffee didn't cure headaches but caused them. Other studies showed that coffee was linked to impotence and even premature death.

Outside Influences

We must remember that any medical study done was influenced by the political and social leaders of the time, and perhaps this is true to this day. There is always one side that will gain from a negative report on caffeine and another who will lose, and these wins and losses in the financial arena can mean billions of dollars. This being so, it would be naive to believe that the influences of these two opposing sides are not in some respects responsible for affecting the outcome of any study on the effects of caffeine.

The Muslims passed on to the Europeans the many medical controversies surrounding coffee and its effects. There was a well known physician at the time who said coffee had properties that could account for the overall mental and physical health of a person consuming the beverage.

Few would argue the ability of caffeine to decrease the effects of inebriation and to increase the rate at which a person recovers from a long night of drinking. But some studies conducted contrasting the behavior of one person drinking coffee and another drinking alcoholic beverages seem to have overlooked some obvious differences in the two beverages. It is quite obvious that those not drinking the alcoholic beverages would perform more efficiently throughout the day than those who were more or less inebriated by day's end.   But other effects were less obvious and not discovered until years later.

Sobriety through Coffee

It was in the 1800s that many doctors were devoting more time to the exploration of caffeine and its effects. There were many diseases that doctors felt caffeine might help ameliorate. They said it could cure headaches, improve memory and digestion, and increase alertness, and even prolong life.

One claim even suggested that caffeine could cure alcoholism, or what at the time was referred to as inebriation. They suggested that caffeinated drinks would promote sobriety. Just attend an AA or NA meeting. Ask any newly sober person how much he depends on his coffee, or if you are truly brave enter the local Alanon Club and just try to do away with the coffee pot and you may change your opinion.

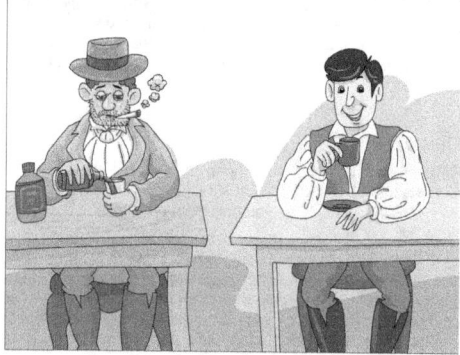

For the sober person who had to face the many social situations that included alcohol, and formerly had little or no alternatives, coffee was truly helpful in maintaining ones sobriety. A sober person who formerly could turn only to alcohol to help soothe his nerves now had a friend in coffee. It served as a social lubricant, and with its popularity it could be found at all the same parties where alcohol was served.

One reason that alcohol consumption was so high during the 1600s was because it was commonly served with every meal; brewing beer was just an everyday part of life for most. It was thought that there was no danger in serving alcohol to children.

Coffee and the Workaholic

The tolerance for this great consumption of alcohol didn't last with the start of the industrial revolution in Europe. The view that drunkenness, and the sloth that it caused, was acceptable quickly vanished. Coffee not only helped the sober stay that way but it helped to lessen alcohol consumption throughout the land and resulted in helping workers maintain performance throughout the day.

In the Western World coffee was vastly popular during the 17th century, and like Europe, coffee became a much better (for the individual and society) morning drink than beer was. One writer of the 1700s noted how coffee should be considered useful in

time management and for the health of those working away under the midnight oil. One can assume from his writing that he understood coffee's ability to boost ones energy and help to fight off tiredness. There was little understanding that using any stimulant could drive one to becoming a workaholic and was thus potentially dangerous.

Historians as well as poets and philosophers wrote of Europeans being saved from the ravages of alcohol by coffee's ability to enhance ones mental state. They wrote that the contrast between the pre-coffee Europe and the post was astounding. It was reported that the European youths, who just fifty years prior had been wildly out of control and frequenting pubs, were now under the good influence of coffee. Coffee was credited with being a nourishing food for the mind and hailed for its ability to heighten rather than weaken ones senses.

Early Claims for Coffee and Tea

A German physician, Leonhard Rauwolf, spoke of his time spent in the East during the 16th century. In his notes he talks directly about coffee, which he refers to as chaube. He tells his readers that in many shops people sat on the floor and partook in this beverage as well as other liquors.

He spoke about people sitting in circles and passing the drink around, taking tiny sips due to the extreme temperatures at which it was served. The physician said the berries and the drink were very common in the cafes. He traveled throughout the eastern world and tells many tales in his memoirs that were read in the west. Some of his experiences were in Persia, where again he wrote about the numerous shops where coffee was being sold and enjoyed.

The medical professionals had high regard for this German physician and tried to apply his principles to all aspects of their studies on caffeine. He spoke of several attributes of coffee - humeral, energizer of body and spirit, cure for headache, stomach ails, and digestion - and doctors of the time blindly followed his lead. They even praised characteristic of coffee when there was no real basis in reality for this.

Perhaps afraid to speak against what the famous physician was reporting, many in the medical field were no longer objective in their studies. It seemed the effects that they were ascribing to coffee were as far-fetched as the idea that the drink served by Helen was merely coffee.

There were suggestions that coffee could cure almost any ailment as well as solving emotional disturbances. There were suddenly many new doctors and experts on tea, coffee, and chocolate, claiming coffee to be the cure all. Around this time, coffee was sold like other drugs and cures, out of apothecaries.

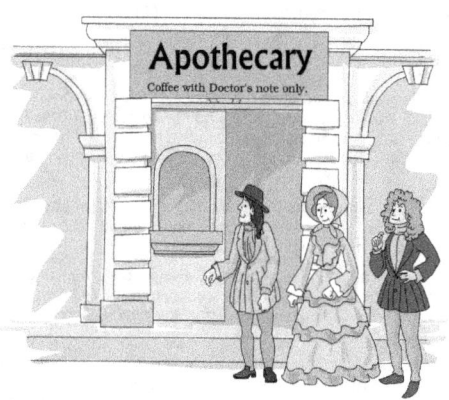

On the Negative Findings

One German physician, Dr. Simon Pauli, was not afraid to disagree with these claims. In a book published in the 17th century he wrote about the negative effects that were caused by the consumption of coffee, chocolate, and tea. He was the primary physician for Dutch royals, and when his works were later read by the Western World his defamation of the three caffeinated beverages became well known.

The first chapter of his book accused the Chinese people of being negligent in their reports on the positive effects of tea, and he stated there were very few if any positive benefits from using coffee or tea.

He suggested that the previous claims of caffeine's ability to cure headaches, stomach ails, and digestion were myths, while its dangers were serious and true. He went so far as to warn its users that they could ultimately die from drinking it. His reports suggested caffeine was especially harmful for those in the middle age group. He saw his role - as one who warned of the dangerous effects of caffeine use - as virtuous and significant to the people.

The Netherlands Welcomes Caffeine

When caffeine was introduced to the Dutch they welcomed it with open arms. There was never any controversy over its use. There were no movements to moderate or abolish it. Doctors and chemists alike were excited about the discovery, and unlike those in other countries they held a positive view on the use of coffee, tea, and chocolate.

One famous chemist and doctor of the 16th century taught that tea could be used to purify the body and was as effective as other remedies used at the time. Another renowned doctor of the 17th century hailed tea's benefits in a medical journal. He recognized early on some of the effects caffeine had that we acknowledge today. This chemist suggested like those before him that it could cure indigestion, headaches, and other illnesses. He documented as well that tea served to help its users fight off sleep and advocated its use for people who needed to stay up all hours of the night for various vocational or religious reasons.

One of the most famous Dutch physicians, who was responsible for the science of chemistry, agreed with his fellow doctors' reports and went on to acclaim the use of caffeine as a blood thinner. Following suit, many doctors began to prescribe high doses of caffeine for indigestion and blood purification, and this was taught in local colleges and universities.

The most influential report though came from a physician near the end of the 17th century, a well known opponent of the physicians in Europe who opposed to caffeine. He was a business man as well as an outspoken physician and was rumored to have opened one of the first German coffeehouses. His promotion of coffee and tea had more influence than any of the other proponents.

He advised that people should start by drinking several cups of tea daily until they could drink as much as they could possibly hold. There are records that actually show he was paid a large sum of money by The Dutch East Indies Trading Company for his praising of tea. It has been established that the trading company hired both scientists and doctors to write favorable reviews of the caffeinated beverages in the hopes that doing so would increase sales. This trend of biased science continues today, having begun hundreds of years earlier in the East.

As Berlin lay in ruins following the end of the Thirty Years War, the Industrial world was in upheaval. Frederick, the king of Germany, trusted the Dutch and felt they had character that was honorable and admirable. He began efforts to take his country out of ruin by appealing to scholars and other worldly men to come to his country. To his credit he was able to lure the famous Dutch physician, Dr. Buntekuh, who had so hailed caffeine in his homeland, to relocate to Germany.

The physician began teaching in universities the same lessons on caffeine he had taught in Europe. He told of the effects of coffee and tea, acknowledging the same characteristics the Europeans already knew about. He was especially excited when speaking about the ability of caffeine to boost vitality. He was one of the greatest advocates of the 1600s for the use of caffeine.

Doctor Buntekuh would go on to publish one of the earliest descriptions of the cacao tree and how its pods were part of the plants unique characteristics. Even though there were such efforts to thrust caffeine upon German society, it would be many years after his death that Germany would be ready to fully embrace coffee.

Disagreement in France

In the late 1600s coffee had finally become available to all classes in France. However, in Paris it still remained affordable only to the royals, and even their supply was limited. In the middle of the 17th century some merchants outside of Paris began to import coffee from the East. It didn't take long before larger imports from Egypt and Lyon began to arrive. Coffee then became a regular part of life in the smaller towns. The first coffeehouse opened outside of Paris and was

37

hugely successful, so much so that shortly after many others were launched and they were equally successful.

There are reports that these early coffeehouses were so popular that they began to spring up all along the countryside. People were drinking coffee in their homes as well. The local merchants, along with the pharmaceutical community, began to import coffee for commercial use. What we seem to recognize in these early experiences is that once something new is well received by the general public there are those who perhaps for personal interest seem to become fearful. This fear tends to turn into anger and is met with equal anger on the side of those embracing the new. This is an age old battle that began as coffee grew in popularity and some doctors found reason to be concerned.

The Same Fight Again

The great debates began again and they were essentially for the same concerns that other countries had argued over for many years before. The stories about caffeine causing upheaval in society and untimely death began again. In France, the physicians, on one hand, tried to spread fear over the possible negative effects of caffeine, citing all manner of diseases that were supposedly caused by its use. Those for the use of coffee were spreading reports of the exaggerated benefits derived from its use. Of course religious society couldn't sit by without putting their two cents in as well. Once again the Islamic physicians brought humeral theories to the table. Towards the end of the 1600s a war of words among the two opposing sides was taking place.

Somewhere in the middle perhaps were the everyday men and women sitting back watching these great debates over a warm cup of coffee. The only party left out until then was local wine merchants who joined the side of those opposed to caffeine, perhaps hoping to maintain their customer base.

An Unpopular Opinion

Towards the end of the 17th century two French physicians ordered a town meeting be held where they sent one of their students to address the city. The audience was made up of other doctors as well as local merchants and the general public. The congregation was told that coffee in other parts of the world had eradicated alcohol, but despite this he felt alcohol was a far superior drug. He told them that coffee was introduced by those hoping to destroy France, and called it impure a drink made by and for savages. He said Europeans had lied about the health benefits of coffee and only did so for self serving purposes.

He said there was no value in coffee's use and that it held no cure for physical or mental ailments. He went on to suggest that because of the way coffee was consumed by the human body it actually caused men to be impotent and suggested it even caused the condition known as palsy.

His talk didn't end there. He also said that coffee was actually made as a cooling beverage and that its energy was responsible for causing both brain and kidney damage by drying up the bodily fluids, including the spinal fluid. The lecturer said it caused problems with urination as well. He suggested that it caused insomnia, where a person's nerves would be destroyed and fatigue. Thereafter, a lack of physical coordination would set in. He attributed coffee with causing excessive leanness and malnutrition. He suggested other theories that coffee can so unbalance the body's fluids that it will eventually destroy every aspect the body - both physical and mental.

The result of this town meeting, and the many reports about the horrible consequence of using coffee, was that doctors were viewed as being egocentric and self serving. Coffee had become so well known and well liked by the time of this meeting that it had little impact whatsoever on the people of France. In fact, the doctors were looked down on and lost respect from these exaggerated reports.

The coffeehouses only became more common and people continued to purchase coffee and consume it in their homes. Despite the physician's best efforts the increased importation of coffee continued from the East. As a result the demand for it continued to grow at rapid speed.

The Ever Changing Medical View of Coffee

There were other physicians that agreed with the views shared in the town meeting. They accepted the findings presented and found it hard to believe that anything other physicians supporting caffeine were saying could be entirely based in fact and thus were skeptical about coffee. As a result most physicians in the late 1600s told their patients to avoid using coffee and suggested to them that it was a lethal and drug of which they should avoid. Soon stories of people overdosing on coffee were spread.

There was a famous business man who was known as a prodigious coffee drinker. When he passed away many rumors about the cause of his death circulated, including tales of coffee poisoning. One exaggerated tale suggested that a well known princess died from coffee poisoning, and there was evidence of this found in her autopsy. The report stated her stomach had many ulcers caused by coffee consumption.

The Scientists Weigh In

Many scientists, though, stood somewhere in the middle of the opposing sides. They didn't believe the exaggerated medical reports about the dangers of coffee. Thus an effort was made among the scientific community at the time to do a controlled, rigid study on coffee. They were hoping to find out the chemical components of coffee and to determine the true nature of each, and whether it was a safe or harmful beverage. Those findings were in direct contrast to those of the medical community. The scientists found that coffee had many benefits.

They saw coffee to be great at warding off drunkenness. They said it cured menstrual cramps as well as stomach problems. The upheld reports that it cured indigestion and was able to help with kidney disease and headaches, along with fighting liver, heart, and lung disease.

They dispelled many reports about how caffeine caused insomnia, and found that coffee was a drug that people should use freely and confidently. Some of these men went on to later write what may be called coffee cookbooks, defending its reputation vigorously. And when contrarian doctors would claim the dangers, the scientist would try to dispel the rumors.

One doctor towards the middle of the 18th century wrote a book that included both the harmful effects as well as the benefits of coffee use. He stated the benefits like helping cure hangovers, curing indigestion, and the stimulation of the mind as well as helping with headaches and memory loss. On the other hand his report included the dangers of coffee use like a decrease in libido and lung disease. In one translation he included the dangers and benefits of chocolate as well.

The Biased Report from the Unbiased Doctor

Dr. Daniel Duncan, working at Montpellier, France, wrote a speech addressing tea, coffee, and chocolate as well as other alcoholic beverages. His memoirs were made public early in the 18th century. They were quite popular and eventually titled "Wholesome Advice against the Abuse of Hot Liquors Particularly of Coffee, Chocolate, Tea, Brandy, and Strong-Waters." Many saw this doctor as a man who didn't jump to conclusions and who was very reasonable so they viewed his book as a valuable resource and it was translated into several languages.

In the first chapters of his book he preached about how there are two sides to everything, neither necessarily being right or wrong, good nor bad. He states that to some degree every person or consumable has both parts.

This author went on to describe the pros and cons of the use of coffee, tea, chocolate and brandy. His view, though more moral than objective, seemed to resemble that of other religious men in that he felt these beverages were to be feared because of how pleasurable they were.

The book makes the same argument that caffeine can be abused, and like other liquors people can become addicted to it and thus avoid other substances that are healthier. He mentions the prevalence of caffeine use in other countries like France to further suggest a society of people addicted to caffeine. It seems his purpose in referring to coffee as liquor is quite obvious. This was his way of placing emphasis on the drug-like quality of coffee.

The author goes on to suggest that the abuse of all three substances was spreading like a plague throughout the land. He said that people of all ages and all classes were suffering from addictions to these beverages. In the end he made an attempt to speak of some of the advantages of coffee, chocolate, and tea. He said that it depended on the person using them and how knowledgeable they were on the effects. He did state that he felt the beverages were not going to kill anyone or save anyone. They were not the toxic poison some claimed them to be, but nor were they the panacea others suggested.

He emphasized that caffeine can be dangerous to people; even if taken in small amounts there can be negative effects. But then goes on to speak of its ability to work as a blood thinner and improve circulation. In the end he concludes that he agrees with others in the medical profession and advises people to be cautious of these liquors.

Despite his cautionary efforts, England is said to have imported more caffeinated product from the end of the 17th century to the middle of the 18th than all the other countries combined. It would seem that though his book was wildly popular few took his advice.

Caffeine and Doctor Harvey

One man who really changed the history of coffee was a professor and physician in England. Dr. William Harvey, who spent much of his life studying coffee in the 16th and 17th century, was one of the most influential men of his time.

He came from a large upper-class family with several siblings who, unlike him, became merchants. The doctor tested well above average as a young boy and was sent to a prestigious school for the gifted. By the time he was in his teens he was already attending medical school. He became fluent in several languages and in his early teens had access to an intellectual world few even know about. By the start of the 17th century he had graduated from medical school and began doing studies abroad. He would later open his medical office in England, and many famous royals along with others mainly in the upper class would be among his patients.

The Father of Modern Scientific Studies

Eventually Dr. Harvey would go on to become one of the founders of scientific medical studies. It was in England where he came up with the theory of caffeine's effect on the blood stream. The university he attended was one of the most well known in the intellectual community and had an international standing While enrolled at this university the doctor made a few discoveries that would change his life and the medical community forever. He was a believer in experimentation and making observations before coming to any conclusions about his subjects of study.

The doctor was the first to discover how coffee affected blood circulation. He discovered that coffee could work as a sort of blood thinner. He was a well known coffee drinker who frequented coffeehouses and had his own stash of imported beans from his travels and studies in the East.

Some suggest that it was a book he read about coffee, which was written by another doctor that may have caught his attention. Other people suggest that on his trip to the East other students encouraged him to try the beverage. The only thing we know for certain is that whatever occurred had a profound effect on the doctor.

After a three year long study abroad Harvey came back to England a changed man. He also returned with some coffee that he recommended to all his colleagues. He would spend the rest of his life promoting the use of coffee, and long after his death he succeeded in changing the way the entire world viewed coffee.

It was at his university that he first became aware of the true effects coffee had on the human body both physically and mentally. He developed a healthy, lifelong obsession with this area of study, and we may be eternally grateful for his efforts.

It was in the early 17th century that Harvey gave his first speech to a group of fellow medical professionals on his favorite subject.

A Well Known Unknown Man

Dr. Harvey was very private in his personal life and there are little details to be found. We do know that he had no children and was married and widowed in his time. One friend spoke of him as an intellectual coffee lover with a nervous energy about him. His friend spoke to his intelligence and his love of coffee that was shared with his siblings. Harvey was in old age by the time the first coffeehouses were being opened, and thus most of his coffee drinking was done at home and in the university.

At the time of his passing those who knew him recalled mainly his love for coffee. He told those close to him that when he died he would hope that his friends would be drinking coffee and celebrating his life. He actually left his belongings, including his coffee beans and pot, to the university he attended.

Unfortunately during his time on earth the doctor's theories were not always well received. There was much speculation and ridicule about his findings. After his death though, upon further investigations, it was found he was ahead of his time in his studies and conclusions.

There is great irony in the fact that this man was well known for his studies on coffee and that without his use of coffee he probably wouldn't have pursued to such a degree. In any case, this man was one who will be remembered throughout time for his love of coffee and his passion for learning and teaching others about the benefits of its use.

In Support of Tea in England

We have already discussed that it was in the 1600s that England was introduced to tea. This can be found in many books by various authors. One poet and medical professional of the time wrote about tea and credited it to helping him stay awake and alert during his night time sessions.

He spoke of the effects it had on him that allowed him not only to stay awake but to be alert enough to do his writing and studying. He described tea as an extraordinary drink that kept him up all night but found him awake and without any negative effects from his lack of sleep. He did say though that only on occasion could he get away with his all night sessions.

More Benefits of Tea

Another Englishman, John Ovington, furthered the work of Dr. Harvey. He claimed tea caused frequent urination and is known to cleanse the body of toxins and help in digestion. In his travels through China he learned that tea was used to treat gout and kidney stones. The Chinese also used tea to cure nausea and increase appetite.

They claimed tea had the wide-ranging ability to enhance ones mental performance, helped sober a person up, increased creativity and treated brain disorders. He spoke of tea's ability to help with circulation and increase physical coordination and strength.

There is a portion of his book where he talks about a person of high intelligence. This person supposedly attributed his own creativity and intellect to his use of tea. Though it remains unknown just what genius he was referring to, perhaps he was erroneously speaking of himself in the third person.

There is one point of view held by this traveling religious man that seems somewhat unique to others of the time. He attributed teas ability to cause insomnia not so much to the caffeine in it, or the stimulation of the body, but more to the stimulation of the mind that it caused.

His focus on this effect of tea makes his story relevant and worth mentioning even though much of his other discoveries were already known. He states that basically if you are ill-tempered or well-humored tea will not really change that characteristic but only enhance it. He claimed that tea will not cure your health if you are really sick. So after many chapters of speaking to the benefits of drinking tea, in the end he put a disclaimer on his earlier findings.

Tea in the Artistic World

In the 17th and 18th century the artistic world created many depictions of tea and coffee. There are poems as well as paintings where the main focal point is the person drinking tea or coffee. Some poetry praises tea and suggests its use by royalty at the time. Others again speak of its ability to inspire and lift ones spirit. One painter at the time claimed that caffeine had a great and lasting impact on his artistic ability.

CHAPTER TWO - COFFEE IN 19ᵀᴴ CENTURY EUROPE

Given enough coffee, I could rule the world. ~Author Unknown

France

In reviewing the medical findings during the first writings about tea and coffee one must remember that the medical community knew nothing about caffeine or its effects One writer in the 19th century, Octave Guelliot, wrote an entire finding on coffee and its addictive nature without ever making mention of the word caffeine. From this forty plus page report not mentioning caffeine we can conclude that it wasn't well known or understood at this time. This writer blames tea and coffee for causing the same list of health problems others attributed to them. He even included a few new ones such as chronic pain in the limbs as well as a change in tongue color, tremors, and sleep disorders.

Guelliot reported that "cafi," which means coffee, was related in nature to drugs like cocaine, alcohol, and morphine. He compared coffee's ability to decrease the appetite and cause fluctuation in body temperature to that of opiates. It might seem outrageous that someone could compare these drugs with the detoxification experiences of coffee users. If you take his report and substitute the word caffeine where the word coffee is used, it may make the claims slightly less outrageous.

He also goes on to give a depiction of how in Europe the use of coffee became so popular. Guelliot spoke of well known writers of the time and tells us that they were addicted to coffee. He talks about how some reports about coffee shortening ones life were essentially disproved when these well-known coffee addicts lived beyond the average life expectancy of the time.

The Beginning of a New Era

This was one of the last writings of the 19th century that contained such little reference of caffeine and its effects. It was after this writing that caffeine would no longer be overlooked in the medical and scientific community. Caffeine was becoming well known, and the effects of caffeine were now attributed to tea and chocolate as well as coffee. So, not long after Guellot published his book it was finally recognized that caffeine was the most active component in tea and coffee.

The Timing of Caffeine's Arrival

For those of us who have come to rely on caffeine for survival in our busy lives it seems unimaginable that those before us seemed to manage just fine without it. It was only in the 1600s Europeans that began to depend on caffeine to help them with the busy work schedules and demands they faced. They depended on caffeine to fight fatigue and to give them just that extra boost they needed. Once they began to thrive with the extra energy and boost that caffeine gave them, it seemed that life simply wouldn't be the same without it.

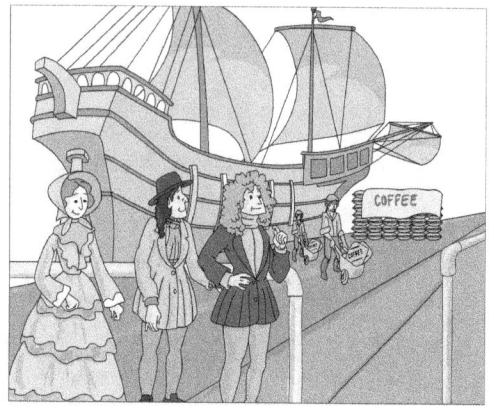

One reason for this new and profound dependence on caffeinated beverages may be linked to the difference in lifestyle prior to its discovery. Men and women of ancient times had relaxed schedules. The work day began when the sun came up and ended essentially when it went down, and there was no need of a beverage that would keep one up all hours of the night. People didn't pay attention to time so much, and until in the 16th century, when time first began to be counted by pendulum, people had much less pressure on them to get things done in the strict time restraints that we face in most parts of the world today.

It would be more than a hundred years later that there was a real accurate clock; and not until the middle of the 17th century was the minute hand in use and accurate. Once the counting of time down to the minute became a way of life, it allowed for a much more accountable society. This introduction of what would eventually become the modern day clock correlated perfectly with the introduction of caffeine in Europe and other places as well.

The New Work Ethic Due to Coffee

The whole new coffee culture was spreading across all of society. Coffee use was on the rise in the literary circles as well as in the scientific community. Coffee was becoming an economic factor as well, having a huge impact on the European trade industry.

Once the impact of a better time measurement really took hold of society it seemed people needed a stimulant to keep up with the pressure. The demands of a much busier lifestyle and action-packed schedules found a society crying out for help. It would seem caffeine arrived on the scene just in time to answer those pleas.

This seemingly perfect combination of time measurement and caffeine had a huge impact on the development of our culture. One of the most important qualities that caffeine had was really what it didn't have. The lack of alcohol in caffeine was greatly appreciated by a society that had suffered much due to the abuse of alcohol. During the early times you must consider that drinking alcohol before and during the work day was a way of life.

Imagine if you can the construction of some of the most famous cathedrals, castles, and bridges in Europe and elsewhere being built by workers who were basically drunk by midday. It is

44

no wonder that many men died during the construction of these buildings and bridges. When one considers just how much alcohol was being drank on a daily basis in the workplace it is no wonder just how welcome the introduction of caffeine really was to government, business, and the church, if not to the population itself.

Caffeine During the Temperance Movement

Caffeine was hailed as a "cure" to those seeking sobriety. It helped men to have a substitute drink they could consume throughout the day that enhanced their productivity rather than detracted from it. Not to mention how it helped people in their ability to show up to work at all. Few are the people who call in to work sick from a caffeine hangover. Suddenly, men who previously showed up to work rarely (and if they did were so intoxicated they could barely function) were now regular and productive. This helped create a much better workforce and allowed for more progess, in many realms, to take place. During the temperance movement caffeine had such a great impact on the industrial world it is hard to really overemphasize it.

There was a tradition at this time to take off at the start of the work week for religious observations. These traditions created a very hectic schedule for the remainder of the week. Also during this revolutionary age there was the introduction of improved machinery that was very expensive. In order to justify the cost of such machinery workers had to work harder and longer.

The harder, longer hours produced much more output and this cycle repeated itself in the industrial world. The more productivity the more money could be invested to purchase machinery that allowed for still higher rates of production. Having sober workers producing considerably more than the previous drunken ones meant they could do much more in shorter periods of time than before. During the 1500s caffeinated beverages underwent a time of experimentation. The taste factor was played with and the result was drinks that were more appealing.

Coffee in the Mini Ice Age

There was at this time a climate change of great proportions taking place. Scientists would look back at the 16th century as the start of a mini ice age in Europe. Hundreds of paintings can be found that depict the gradual increase in size of the glaciers between the 16th and 19th century. There are photographs, paintings, and sketches that depict this ice age taking place beginning around the time caffeine was introduced. During an ice age one can imagine a hot beverage that lifted ones spirits without rendering them incapacitated was more than welcomed.

Some reports from this period tell of the Lower Grindelwald glacier and how people looked to men of religion in the hopes that somehow they could make the glacier retreat. People went so far as to pay the way for a priest to come and perform and exorcism on the land. There was some relief from the glacier for a short period of time, but glacier eventually returned larger than ever and created a freeze that only worsened over time.

During the later part of the 17th century there were famines throughout Europe due to the extremely cold winter. There was snow during summertime in parts of Europe, and eventually the warm seasons shortened and the winters became longer and more brutal.

There are many reasons why the mini ice age may have occurred. The earth is said to have shifted and there was a reduction of solar heat as well as volcanic activity that may have had an impact on the atmosphere. All of these things combined were most likely to blame for the ice age that occurred in Europe.

Europeans at that time turned to coffee for many reasons. One effect of coffee is to lessen the appetite and this was needed in a time of great famine. They also used coffee as a means of keeping warm. Lastly they used coffee in attempt to lift the spirits of the people at that time of hardship. The result of this increase in coffee consumption, and the welcome effects it had on the people of Europe was that as they emerged from the mini ice age, coffee emerged as the most popular drink on earth.

CHAPTER THREE - THE SOCIETAL IMPACT OF TEA & COFFEE

Coffee is to the body what the Word of the Lord is to the soul. - Isak Dinesen

Tea and coffee have much in common when we look back at the history of each. However there are great distinctions made between the two by its users and by those who study the drinks. Coffee has, since its introduction, held a more masculine image. It is often associated with the artistic world. We remember how the bohemian society so welcomed coffee. Coffee is also often associated with those who are more vocal with their feelings about politics, human rights, and not conforming to those in charge. It was always labeled more a drink of the rebellious and boisterous. Coffee was seen more as a drug that people depended on, rather than a social nicety.

We remember from our early discussion that coffee was many times classified with other drugs like alcohol, cocaine, and tobacco. It was labeled as a dangerous drug that could harm a person mentally and physically. It also held an image that its users stay up late and had a tendency to be workaholics.

Tea on the other hand held a more feminine image. Pictures depict women in long dresses drinking tea in drawing rooms out of delicate tea cups. Words like meditation and spirituality are linked with tea even to this day. Tea was the tranquil drink of the elite members of society: a drink made for the elderly and those who were calm and at peace with themselves and with society.

These extremely different depictions of the two drinks can be found from the beginning of the coffeehouse and the tea culture of Japan. Tea houses met with little if any opposition, while coffeehouses faced opposition from all directions.

Coffee was often the subject of bans from kings, law enforcement, and the government throughout time. Tea on the other hand was never to appear on lists of forbidden substances.

Why the Hypocrisy?

As one looks at these very different perceptions of the two drinks, it is quite perplexing in light of the many similarities they share. Consider that each comes from vegetable matter. Coffee and tea both have easily recognizable aromas. Each can be served chilled or heated. Many people use sweeteners and creamers with both. In almost every town on earth you can find both. Coffee and tea both work as stimulants, and each imparts many of the same physical and mental effects on the human body.

While there may be more caffeine in the typical cup of coffee in comparison to the typical cup of tea, the truth is that most people who use tea drink a larger quantity than those who drink coffee, so even this difference is fairly invalid.

Why the Prejudice?

Why is there such a clear distinction made between the two beverages? Why are the two cultures said to be so different? Why is tea considered to be civilized and prestigious in both the

47

East and West, while coffee has never held these titles anywhere in the world? Why is coffee often the victim of exaggerated negative reports in ancient times and still today, while tea has never merited much more than a raised eyebrow throughout time?

Below we will list some of the common characteristics associated with both beverages and the culture of people who drink them. This chart is to give us a clearer picture of the distinctions made.

Characteristics said to be of each:

Coffee/Coffee Drinkers	Tea/Tea Drinkers
Masculine	Proper
Used as vice	Virtuous
Dangerous	Female
Bohemians drink it	Harmonious
Poison	Distinguished
Abuse	Romantic
Frantic	Tranquility
Overwork	Pure
Excessiveness	Relaxation
Yang	Yin

We can look at this chart and see the obvious differences in the words associated with the two beverages and those who drink them. When trying to find the reason for these differences we need only look back and see that they existed since the beginning of caffeine's introduction to the world.

Cola drinks, and other drinks made by carbonization that contain caffeine, have a much shorter history and have not seen the many ups and downs that both coffee and tea have. They are often associated with the younger generation. Most commercials depict the users of cola drinks happy and participate in activities that require more energy. The irony here of course is that with all the other added ingredients in cola drinks we know them to be truly harmful without question.

It is in the East that we see the greatest of distinctions between coffee and tea. Simply look to Japanese works of art and you can see the light in which tea is portrayed. It is often royalty drinking tea, or delicate looking women sitting in a peaceful setting. In Japanese poetry and other literature tea is described with many of the same words we used in our chart.

Drinking tea is considered to embody what it means to be a part of true Japanese culture. Caffeine may have been viewed with some skepticism, but even though tea contained it, the Japanese viewed tea as a wholesome perfect drink. It was not until the 1900s that the coffeehouse was embraced in Japan, but a place mainly for business transactions and for louder social discussions than would happen in the teahouse.

In England, coffee is depicted as being drank by boisterous business men. Even from the beginning of the coffeehouse this depiction was readily accepted. In both countries the two drinks are equally recognized as a part of everyday life though. They are both used on a regular basis in traditional settings and have been since the early days of caffeine. We can also assume that if either drink were suddenly to vanish there would be a public outcry.

Early Days of Coffee in Japan

The first recorded documentation of coffee being consumed in Japan dates back to the 18th century. Coffee was met with a cold reception by the Eastern world. It would take many years

48

before the drink was really accepted there. It was near the end of the 19th century that we can find references to coffee houses being opened.

Early in the 20th century the coffeehouses of the Far East resembled those of the Middle East. Teahouses actually began to import coffee for the purpose of selling it to its patrons.

The same fear that spread in the Islamic world about the coffeehouse and its role in political upheaval occurred in Japan. In the wake of the Second World War the Japanese government closed the coffeehouses.

The bans didn't last though, and by the middle of the 20th century coffee shops and cafes that were already common in the Western countries began to re-emerge in Japanese culture. The coffeehouses of the Far East were really places for businessmen to meet with one another outside the confines of the office.

The Many Styles of Japanese Coffeehouses

There were some coffeehouses geared towards different styles of music. There were jazz coffeehouses and more traditional coffeehouses. These became hangouts for performers and those hoping to someday become performers. They played and continue to play an important role in the music world. These are places where patrons can listen to original pieces of work. Sometimes it is in these very coffeehouses where musicians are discovered, and chance encounters take place to this day that change the music world.

There were coffeehouses that only hired waitresses that were considered to be beautiful. Others were geared towards attracting worldly travelers. Some were geared to be a place where people of different nationalities could meet with one another.

There were also many different things that were sold from these coffeehouses, including breads and pastry items. There were others that sold sandwiches, novelties, and specialty coffees for the home. Coffee was expensive during those days and could cost in the upwards of four to six dollars per cup.

A Coffeehouse for Everyone

Shortly after WWII, there were hundreds of coffeehouses and cafes in Japan. Japanese society was forever changed as a result. Many Japanese homes were tiny and the coffeehouse was a place where people could socialize with friends and colleagues without the tight confines. The expense of the drink was well worth the opportunity that was found in being able to socialize in these coffeehouses and cafes.

In the early 20th century there was finally a break in the cost of coffee and coffeehouse chains began to sell coffee much cheaper, to where today it is around two dollars a cup. There was one popular coffeehouse chain that had more than 500 outlets, but as you can imagine they found competition with the Seattle-based Starbucks that soon opened in Japan. Starbucks was seen as a brand new concept in the coffeehouse tradition. Starbucks was given all the rave reviews that it received in the Western World, but really the same could be and was said about the coffee culture everywhere.

Japanese coffeehouses were unique in the amount of diverse cultures they appealed to. One could find a coffeehouse that attracted virtually all lifestyles with little trouble. Today in Japan there are over one hundred thousand coffeehouses. In Tokyo alone there are over sixteen thousand.

The coffeehouses themselves are works of art. In some Japanese coffeehouses, which are many stories high, the artwork inside is often original masterpieces.

The internet is as common as the coffee in most coffeehouses in Japan. The reason for this may be that the original role of the coffeehouse in Japan was to serve the businessman. In Japanese culture, much like in the Western World, the internet is an integral part of everyday business.

The Japanese were the pioneers in accommodating patrons' needs. Many other Asian countries copied Japan, and cybercafés can be found everywhere today. Places like Hong Kong and Korea copied Japan in many other ways as well. They offer patrons the chance to sit outdoors and listen to live music while enjoying their coffee. These types of coffeehouses can actually be traced back to the early Islamic nations.

Specialty Coffee

Japanese culture will always be linked with the use of tea, but you may be surprised to learn that coffee has supplanted tea as the drink of choice. Many people argue that the Japanese actually have more flavors and higher caffeinated coffee than can be found in the Western World. But we still hold the title for making specialty coffees that taste the best.

Despite the popularity of coffee in Japan, the average household doesn't brew its coffee at home or even have the means to. The culture is changing and with it this tendency will most likely change as well.

England and the Early Coffeehouses

It is unclear precisely when tea, coffee, and chocolate became popular in England. There are quotes by Shakespeare in the 16th and 17th century that relate to almost all aspects of everyday life. Shakespeare was known to comment on the favored food and beverages of his time. It is the lack of any mention of coffee in his work that lead one to believe it was not until after his time that coffee, tea, and chocolate were well known in England.

Sir Frances Bacon wrote a few years after Shakespeare's death about coffee, which he referenced only a few times. From what we know about coffee in his time, we can assume his references to the beverage were more third person than first hand experiences. At that time coffee had to be prescribed from ones physician. Ironically Dr. William Harvey was said to have been his doctor.

The Little Coffeehouse that Could

Much of the writings of coffee at the time were not firsthand accounts. A fellow named Aubry did many personal interviews. He was not a popular man but still is credited with being one of the first to offer a history of the early coffeehouses in England. He tells of an instance where a Lebanese Jew, Cirques Jacob, traveling from the East to England was given a stash of coffee beans and told how to use them. It is said that another Jew later in the same year opened his own coffeehouse.

This man was also from the East and was said to have sold coffee as well as chocolate. Chocolate was becoming quite desirable in England at this time and the Easterner was willing to cash in. His coffeehouse remained open for another decade and then was sold again and remained open as a restaurant for hundreds of years.

The Coffeehouse Takes the Blame

In just a few years coffeehouse were opening all over England. There were some who looked upon this development as a detriment to society. The view from these men was that the coffeehouse was actually a threat to the intellectual society. This opinion was shared by many who looked to the gossip taking place in these coffeehouses and found reason for concern. In the 17th century there were those who blamed the problems facing English culture on the coffeehouse. They felt that men were wasting their time in coffeehouses much as they had in pubs. They were sitting around talking politics rather than taking an active role in changing matters. There were those who once held roles of ministry in the church who were now just spending their time talking of worldly matters in the coffeehouse.

The spread of this opinion would result in university leaders encouraging students and faculty to refrain from becoming a part of the coffeehouse culture. Towards the end of the 17th century there was a ban on coffee being sold on Sunday evenings. This ban is much the same as bans of today on alcoholic substances in some Western cities. At one point they tried to completely close coffeehouses on Sundays.

However, once more, these efforts proved useless in curtailing the use of coffee. The popularity of coffee only grew as did the number of coffeehouses opening throughout England.

University Life and the Coffeehouse

There was then and to this day great rivalries between English colleges and universities. Reports from the 17th century suggest that the coffeehouse was the popular hangout for students. There was one coffeehouse that served as the site for a local newsletter, and conversation inspired by coffee became the fodder. The coffeehouses became extremely popular, so much so that again those in charge tried to regulate them. There was a statute that made it equally punishable for students to be caught entering a coffeehouse as it was for them to be caught in a pub. But as with all those before it, these efforts to control peoples' coffee consumption failed.

By the 18th century the success of the coffeehouse to lure students throughout England saw no end in sight. At this time it became just as common for one to find the professors and other faculty at the local coffeehouse as the students. All subjects were discussed at the local coffeehouse by students and faculty alike.

The Coffee Club

There is a story about a man who was persuaded by local students to sell coffee from his home. They formed a club that met regularly in the man's home to discuss the troubles of the world over a cup of coffee. Eventually this small meeting of students would become the Oxford Coffee Club, a society that leads the world in scientific studies to this day. They were studying caffeine, which at the time was a drug that few knew much about. The notes from these early meetings suggest that those attending drank coffee in large quantities, not merely for its taste but more to study and understand the effects of doing so.

Some that were members of the club were less interested in the experiments the members were conducting. These members were more interested in the social opportunities that being a part of the exclusive club granted. Some of the early members were astronomers, physicists, artists and other well known men of science.

Famous Members

The group had become a science club and a well known. The first participants included Hans Sloane, founder of the British Museum, Sir Edmund Halley, the great astronomer, and Sir Isaac Newton.

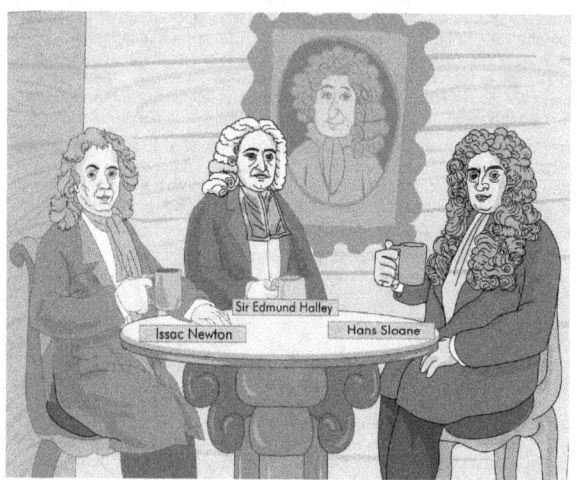

Sir Edmund Halley

Issac Newton

Hans Sloane

Sloane was responsible for many others joining the club. This coffee club began traveling and sharing their studies with other clubs throughout England. Some labeled the members more as philosophers than scientists. They perceived the "studies" to also be less scientific and more philosophical in nature. But as word of the many hands-on experiments taking place in these clubs spread, so did their popularity.

By the 17th century these clubs had become mini universities, and many of the graduates went on to be famous in a broad variety of fields. Some members would later become distinguished professors and university leaders. There were famous architects, astronomers, writers, poets, inventors and physicians that attended these clubs in their university days.

It was the Oxford Coffee Club that was said to host the highest intellectuals of the time. There were meetings held nightly and political writers of the time often made reference to the coffeehouse and the coffee club. These meetings and the things discussed at them became a part of literary history.

Some coffeehouses at that time served alcoholic beverages as well. It was a time when the consumption of caffeinated beverages was taken into peoples' homes as well. An advertisement from the 17th century for the sale of tea, chocolate, and coffee also offered instruction on how to prepare them.

Sober Hang Outs

In the middle part of the 17th century coffeehouses were opened all over Europe. Coffee was being hailed as a cure for alcoholism. They were credited in with maintaining sobriety in society. As a result, many who usually hung out in the local taverns or on the streets were now gathering in large numbers at the coffeehouses. These people, who were often seen as the transient members of society, did nothing to help the reputation of the coffeehouse. The original coffeehouse went through changes at this time and many of those changes were unwelcome and attributed to the new class of people flocking to them as a means of staying sober.

At the later part of 17th century women were not allowed in coffeehouses, and this served as another reason for disapproval from the masses. One unhappy wife began a petition to make coffee itself forbidden. She went so far as to blame coffee as the reason for her husband's impotence. She went on to suggest that society at large was in danger because of the beverages impact on the marital bed.

Other angry wives referred to themselves as coffeehouse widows, suggesting their domestic partnerships were being endangered as husbands stopped by the coffeehouse on the way home from a hard day of work and didn't return until the wee morning hours. In response, the King proclaimed a ban on coffeehouses.

The Men Answer Back

Don't be mistaken that the men didn't take this attack on their beloved coffeehouses lying down. They got together and wrote a pamphlet of their own defending their coffee use. That was followed by a book with illustrations that hailed the use of coffee. This book was sold upon the opening of a coffee mill specializing in the sale of Arabian coffee and chocolate.

More exaggerated tales spoke about how men were being led astray by the coffeehouse, led into meaningless conversations with strangers, causing them to slack in their work lives as well as their personal lives. The report went on to say that men spent hour upon hour at the coffeehouses discussing nonsense and their reputations suffered greatly.

There were other serious claims as well. The report suggested that the economy was also suffering as a result of the coffeehouses and coffee sales. They suggested that farmers were facing ruin as they saw loss in their sale of oats, wheat, and other products. Thus as farmers were going out of business, the impact on those who depended on rents also suffered.

This report suggested that coffee was responsible for a great time of suffering in the country, all of which could be linked to the coffee bean.

A Coffeehouse Here, a Coffeehouse There

In the 1600s many of the England coffeehouses were beginning to imitate the tradition set forth by the Japanese. They began to create the coffeehouse around the culture. There were coffeehouses that catered to poets and musicians. There were coffeehouses geared towards the business man and merchants. There is no concrete proof of the exact number of coffeehouses, but it appears in several accounts of the time that there were hundreds.

From several sources, including tax records as well as genealogy, it is estimated that the population in England at the time was around five million. Some of the bigger cities had populations in the hundreds of thousands. These estimates vary throughout literature but are considered to be fairly accurate.

The popularity of the coffeehouse in the 17th century led to many exaggerated reports that there were several thousand coffeehouses in the bigger cities alone. This report can be found in many writings. One writer concluded that there were as many coffeehouses in Europe as there were in Egypt. Certainly he said that for every profession and every hobby a man may have, he could find a coffeehouse in England catering to that particular interest.

Many books of the time spoke of the popularity of the coffeehouse and the alarming number of them in Europe. Yet another book suggests that in the 18th century there were hundreds not thousands of coffeehouses.

When comparing these estimates to modern day numbers it seems they are exaggerated, but it is hard to really determine for sure either way. Today in the west, by comparison, there are more than ten thousand coffeehouses in the entire nation. Even in bigger cities like New York City there are not as many coffeehouses today as there were reported to have been in the biggest cities of England. This would mean that in England there were over thirty times as many coffeehouses as there are in all of New York today. This seems obviously illogical.

In the 19th century, coffeehouses in England underwent a rapid decline. In less than two hundred years England saw the rise and fall of the coffeehouse. Today in the largest city in England there are only dozens of coffeehouses, not hundreds. Despite the rapid decline in the amount of coffeehouses there has been a steady increase in the use of caffeinated products, and the influence of the coffeehouse in England can still be seen every day in all of society.

Caffeine and Royalty

There is a long and complicated history between caffeine and royalty as well as others in authority. Many attempts at banning the use of caffeine, along with the places where it was sold, have occurred throughout time. Ironically, records at the time indicate that royalty often drank and served caffeinated beverages in their kingdoms.

Here is another area where we see the contrast in how coffee and tea were viewed differently. The Queen could be found serving tea in her tea room while the King was giving orders to ban coffee throughout the land. In the 17th century coffeehouses were banned altogether in parts of England. This was a time when the popular opinion on coffee shifted, and again it was looked at with paranoia.

The King ruled that coffeehouses created a society of apathetic people. He said that the industrial world had suffered much, as men no longer were concerned with their employment but spent all their time in coffeehouses.

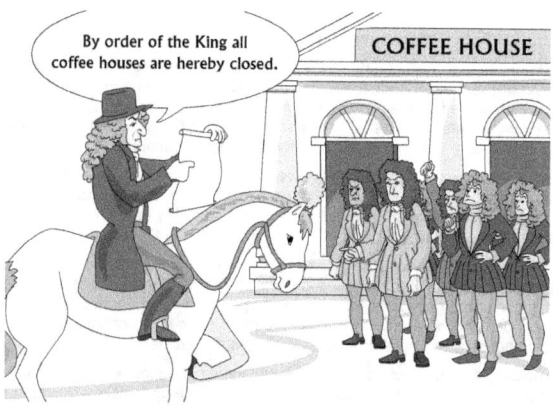

The King also stated that the conversations held in the coffeehouses were against the government. All types of evil were said to being plotted in these establishments, and lies being spread about the Kingdom. He called the coffeehouses both evil and filled with danger. The result from all these accusations was that as of December 29, 1675, the people of England were strictly banned from even entering any establishment serving coffee. They were called "seminaries of sedition." And the people were warned against purchasing coffee and even against using it in their homes. The ban included tea as well as chocolate.

Most stoves at that time had open flames and one theory suggests that one reason for these strict bans had to with a fear of the fire hazard posed by boiling water for these drinks. There had been a huge and devastating fire not many years before this time. Certainly the main reason, though, lay in the King's fear of social revolution that could stem from the social gatherings that were taking place. His reasons were so similar to those of sultans and others in authoritative roles that it cannot be discounted.

Those who were following the bans on coffee throughout the world saw these similarities and spoke of them in their writings. The King also tried to force his people to strictly follow religious practices and used this as reason for the ban on coffeehouses. Perhaps it was reports coming back to him from the people who suspected his bans were for much more self-serving purposes than the King suggested they were.

This 17th century ban was even shorter than others had been, as the people voiced a loud outcry. The nation of coffee drinkers and coffeehouse owners were disgusted by the Kings ban and this, along with the economic effect of the ban, seemed to be enough for the King to withdraw his decree after less than two weeks.

The King had lost some support for his ban as people saw it as a measure that had been blindly taken, and was entirely self-serving in nature. Many of the King's men frequented the coffeehouses, and they were able to discuss more freely what was going on in England from their perspectives.

One reason many question whether the King was really as serious as he claimed to be with his ban is the great amount of revenue he collected from those taxes on caffeinated beverages. These were taxes the King couldn't justify cutting off. He relied heavily upon this revenue, and abolishing the drinks from which they came simply wouldn't have been a reasonable decision.

Tea Takes Over

One of the first coffeehouses in England in the 17th century sold tea as well. It stated many of the virtues of tea as being an entertaining drink that worked as a therapeutic beverage. In attempts to gain customers, they appealed to the fine reputation that it had. Tea was served alongside with coffee and chocolate. Tea became just as popular in England as it was in the Eastern World. Tea seemed to curb the countries appetite for alcoholic beverages much like coffee had.

The new Queen, wife of Charles II, helped England undergo a facelift of sorts. She was a very rich woman before entering into marriage. She introduced culture to the realm in the form of the finest of imports, including spices and different fabrics like silk. She brought gems and jewelry from her travels around the world. Thus, in time the country became acclimated to the more luxurious lifestyle set forth by the Royals. Tea was well known at this time by the richer members of society.

Part of the Queen's wedding gift was a huge supply of tea. It took little time for society to look to her and to follow in her footsteps, and thus tea became a popular drink amongst all of society. The country had acquired an outlet that allowed them to access the many spoils of India, which beforehand they couldn't do. This acquirement had a huge impact on society as with it came many spoils.

The Queen was a great advocate for drinking tea and she also introduced sugar into daily life for the people. Sugar became one of the most profitable revenue sources of the time.

There came into being many new ways of preparing tea. One author talks about how a Jesuit missionary, returning from his travels to the East, found a way to make tea that required the use of egg yolks. He hailed this drink as a cure for hunger and to settle nausea and cleanse the blood.

The tea movement in England only grew stronger after the death of Charles II died; and the Queen, who first introduced tea to mainstream society, returned to her homeland. The next Queen, Mary, had a love affair with tea as well, and felt it was a required part of the prestigious circles in which she traveled. She had a tea table that became the newest quest for her imitators to acquire. The ladies of high society were all drinking tea and collecting the many things that having the proper tea party required. These traditions continued even after Mary's sister, Anne, took the throne.

Ladies were meeting on a regular basis to gossip over tea and to go in search of the latest necessity, whether that a rosewood tea table or ivory tea cups, it was deemed important to have these items.

One writer of the period, known to be a tea consumer, spoke of a meeting with the Queen in which he says they drank cup after cup all day long. He said few words were spoken but many cups were consumed.

The practice of having a late afternoon tea session didn't actually begin until the 19th century. The reason for the delay was that beer was still considered a morning beverage and it took some time for tea to overtake it as the more preferred breakfast drink. However, by the 18th century there were reports of tea starting to become the common breakfast beverage.

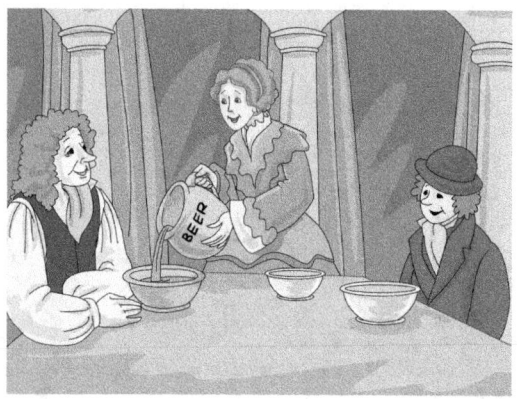

CHAPTER FOUR – THE FIGHT FOR THE RIGHT TO CAFFEINATE

Chocolate, men, coffee - some things are better rich. ~Author Unknown

Coffee comes to America

The man who is credited with first introducing coffee to the continent of North America was also the founder of Virginia. Captain John Smith learned of coffee on his travels abroad. There are no reports that any of the first settlers in the New World in the early parts of the 17th century had any caffeinated belongings with them on their voyages. Some say it was the Dutch and the British who were the first to introduce tea and coffee to the new colonies. It was near the latter part of the 17th century that the first documented reference to the presence of coffee was made. In New York the drink was known, as was the process of brewing coffee beans. We can find references to spices being used with coffee as well at this time.

Before the introduction of coffee and caffeinated beverages in North America, beer was the common morning drink. Much like in England and other places coffee was a welcome addition to the morning of most Americans.

We can also look at records that indicate, around this same period, chocolate was being used for its medicinal qualities. Coffee cost around four dollars a pound at that time and was considered to be quite expensive. Some reports state that the price for one small cup of coffee was about the same as a meal would have cost.

Due to the cost of caffeinated beverages, alcoholic drinks were still more popular with meals. Tea was slightly less expensive and found to be served more often than chocolate or coffee.

The First American Coffeehouse

The first coffeehouse of North America can be traced back to Massachusetts. It had the same name as the well known English coffeehouse: "London Coffeehouse". It became the place where the first known license to sell coffee to the public was acquired.

This same coffeehouse is still open today, but is now a well known café that sells books as well as caffeinated beverages. Many famous authors are said to have sold books there.

This combination of coffeehouse and book shop can be dated back to the middle of the 17th century in England. As we discussed in earlier, there are magazines as well as newspapers that were actually printed and sold from the coffeehouses. America upheld this tradition as well.

At the end of the 17th century the King's Arms coffeehouse opened in New York. Stories about this coffeehouse refer more to the outward appearance than the coffee drank inside. It was said to be bright in color and it had a great view to the rest of the city. This famous coffeehouse was actually purchased abroad and then shipped to the colonies piece by piece.

The next coffeehouse to open in the east, in Philadelphia, is said to have been the only functioning structure in the city at that time (acting as a post office), and thus became well known to the people. There is mention of the famed "Ye Coffeehouse" in a well known newspaper of the time, referring to the excellent coffee that was sold by the printer, Benjamin Franklin.

The next coffeehouse to follow suit was started by a man already in the publishing field. William Bradford's version of the London Coffeehouse became a well known place to conduct business. There were many different transactions occurring in this mid 18th century coffeehouse. It became a marketing place for anything from coffee beans to slaves. There were men of all walks of life going in and out of the coffeehouse on a regular basis.

The English tradition of coffeehouses becoming the new hang out for college and university students continued in America. Coffeehouses were becoming common, and just as common were the meetings that students were holding in them. They may have been quite popular among the young classmates due to the other beverages being sold. During the early days coffeehouses sold alcoholic beverages along with the coffee. Though they may have gotten the idea from the English, what happened in America from these meetings went beyond anything the English had ever seen.

The Revolution and the Coffeehouse

The meetings that began with one or two university students discussing politics over coffee and beer soon became official sites for trials and city council meetings. One well known coffeehouse, "The Green Dragon," towards the end of the 17th century, served the most famous of American rebels including Paul Revere and John Adams.

This coffeehouse served as a tavern and inn as well, and in many places in American literature it has been referred to as playing an important role in the Revolution.

Many soldiers and men in government, as well as other royalty, met in this famed coffeehouse plotting seditious acts. It is rumored that men who were part of the greatest revolutions of the time, including the Boston Tea Party and the Masonic Movement, met in this same coffeehouse.

The Tea Tax

The relationship between the Boston Tea Party and Americans love affair with tea and coffee intersected in 1773. Americans, facing excessive taxes that made tea too expensive for most, eventually revolted against the British. This act of dumping the containers of tea into the ocean changed history.

It was at this very time that Americans turned to coffee as the more popular drink. Prior to the taxes on tea in the 18th century, tea and coffee were both equally enjoyed by most in America. Remember also that this revolutionary act was conspired in the back rooms of coffeehouses. It was at the Green Dragon where Paul Revere and others supposedly planned the Boston Tea Party.

Coffee, from that moment in time until today, became the more popular drink at breakfast. Few people know American history well enough to be aware that it was at a coffeehouse that the Declaration of Independence was first read publicly. This makes it hard to deny the influence that coffee has had on American culture.

Another revolution was taking place in a coffeehouse located in New York City. It was at the New York Merchant's Coffeehouse where that the Sons of Liberty met in the 18th century to draft the First Continental Congress.

This coffeehouse played an important part of celebrating the victories of war. Washington himself was celebrated here after his election. The stories of how many important meetings - that changed the course of American history took place in coffeehouses - can be found throughout American literature.

One point that can also be made when we look back at American history is that perhaps the early "paranoia" of other countries was well founded. Many Kings and other leaders around the world feared the coffeehouse would become a place where revolutions against the government were born. In America, during the 18th and 19th Centuries, this proved to be the case.

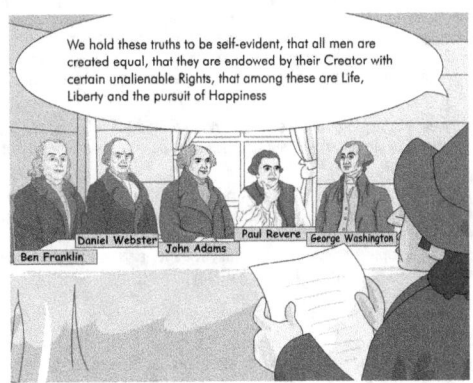

The Most Expensive Coffeehouse

One coffeehouse, built at the start of the 19th century, cost nearly half a million dollars. This was unheard of at that time. The coffeehouse was many stories high and nothing was too luxurious when it came to the inside and the outside. It was modeled after Lloyd's of London and became a popular hangout for the well to do in the import export business.

The coffeehouse was designed by one of the most famous American architects of all time. It was the host for many extravagant banquets and celebrations. The guest lists would impress anyone interested in American history. It was the most expensive coffeehouse ever opened to date but burned down only a few years after its opening.

Alcoholism and Coffee: Take Two

The early days of American coffeehouses were times of heavy alcohol drinking both in England and the colonies. During the early 18th century there was a problem with alcoholism ravaging cities on both sides of the Atlantic. We can see from the descriptions of children born to alcoholic women during that time that fetal alcohol syndrome as we now know it was occurring in America and in other places as well.

During this period the highest alcohol consumption rates ever recorded took place. By the later part of the 18th century physicians were pleading for help with the problem and calling for awareness. Some doctors began campaigns to end alcohol use entirely while others advocated moderation. One doctor, Benjamin Rush, was publishing books that advocated the use of caffeinated beverages to help fight the ravages of alcohol. He had many who supported his cause and his books sold by the thousands. Though his efforts definitely increased the consumption of caffeinated beverages, they did little to curb the consumption of alcohol at that time.

Coffee in the 19th Century

In the later part of the 1800s America had the highest coffee consumption rates of any country. Americans viewed themselves as more down to earth and more pioneering a people than the English. The English were seen by many as more snobbish and delicate. Americans were proud of their coffee consumption and welcomed the title as the nation consuming the most of the beverage. In one of Twain's famous writings he refers to coffee both in America and across the world. He said that European coffee was so weak and unpleasant that it made American coffee the standard bearer.

In most references Twain makes, he speaks of American coffee in high regard. He leaves one with the image that he suffered while having to spend time abroad in regards to the coffee he had to drink.

Twain's words were so inspiring that to this day Americans will argue anyone who suggests that European coffee is equal in taste to American. Despite his bleak view of foreign coffee, Twain appears to have embraced the tea of other countries. He paints the picture of tea being an inspiring drink that awakened people bored with their daily routine, and made them see the beauty of the world around them as they enjoyed a cup of tea at day's end.

America's Coffee Revolution

America was enjoying a time of being not just the World leader in industry but also one of the richest countries in the World. The America was a melting pot of different cultures and belief systems coexisting amongst one another. Naturally, due to their role as a political, military, and education power in the 1900s, the Americans viewed themselves as the experts on caffeine.

One feature common in almost every American coffeehouse was the free refill. This was in sharp contrast to European coffeehouses where the cost of one cup was almost double the price. There were no free refills in Europe either; in fact the cups were considerably smaller. This was the only thing about American coffee that really impressed the European visitors when they came to America.

The story of caffeine in America owes much to the cultural love affair with coffee. One can assume that the affordable cost and the free refill had much to do with Americans warm embrace of their beloved drink. Since the Boston Tea Party, America has been the largest importer of coffee with no other nation close to them in that title. Coffee is responsible for more than half of the caffeine consumption in the United States.

Coffeehouses had a history of hosting poetry readings and musical sessions dating back to the first coffeehouses in the 1500s. They have long been the home to travelers and the artistic bohemian culture. In the United States, the artistic movement in coffeehouses began in the med-20th century. The coffeehouse became a popular place for the Hippie generation to hang their hats all across the country. Previously it had been the beatnik generation. These movements began in California and quickly spread east, having a great impact on the image of the coffeehouse as a place for those less reputable to frequent.

During the beatnik generation there were many famous poets who held readings encouraging the spirit of experimentation and independent thinking. One common theme among these poets and songwriters was the use of drugs and alcohol. This theme was taken further and to much higher levels during the hippie generation that followed. The poets and songwriters of both these generations were more than willing to talk about their own drug and alcohol use, and they glorified it as a means of finding truth and freedom.

Some of the most famous musicians of our time found their starts performing in front of live audiences in coffeehouses. The music of the hippie movement was often times very political in nature. Neil Young was one of those musicians who spoke against the war and challenged his listeners to be independent thinkers, and not to blindly follow those in power. Young was infamous for his anti-war lyrics. One can Google Neil Young; and it doesn't take long to find the word coffeehouse strongly associated with his performances.

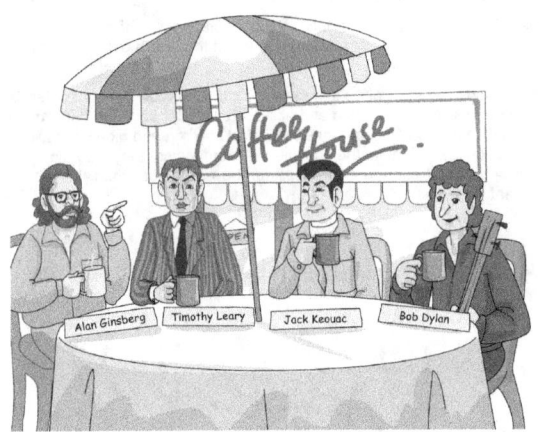

The 20th century has seen the growth of the coffeehouse in America like no other era. There are many chain coffeehouses like Starbucks, The Coffee Bean, and Tully's. These are just a few of many chain coffeehouses that can be found in nearly every American city. This doesn't speak to the cafes and bookstores that have also geared their business to suit the coffee addicts of America. Today, in many cities, even the local grocery stores have a coffee shop of some kind in them. Some of these coffeehouses have drive-through windows and are open all hours of the morning and night to meet the needs of the American coffee culture. A few of the traditional coffeehouses turned away from development for a period of time only to come back stronger than ever, opening more coffeehouses and cafes as they saw others doing with great success.

Soft Drinks Meet Hard Opposition

Tea and coffee were always recognized first as drugs, and then later for their quality as a pleasurable drink. The first colas were also seen as drugs and they were sold much in the same way cold medicine is sold today at drug stores. By the beginning of the 20th century, Coca-Cola became a well-known and well-liked drink. Facing many adverse reactions by the public for its rumored cocaine content, the Coca-Cola company had to overcome adversity just like tea and coffee had in their beginnings. The company denies that cocaine was ever an ingredient. However the caffeine content in the drink, then and now, is still met with disapproval, even though the caffeine content was cut in half.

Coca-Cola and the Man Who Tried To Banish It

A well known, powerful physician of the late 19th and early 20th century spoke out vehemently against Coca-Cola. Dr. Harvey Wiley almost succeeded in destroying the entire company with his reports. His role was to protect society from any dangerous components in their food and drink. He was a well-respected man and he was appalled at the way the nation so eagerly embraced and indulged in the use of caffeinated beverages.

He especially frowned upon the use of caffeinated soft drinks as they were more geared towards the youth. The doctor was greatly alarmed about the health of the younger generation in respect to their caffeine consumption.

He saw the obvious fact that coffee and tea were consumed almost exclusively by adults. He also stated that adults were well informed and able to truly understand the consequences of caffeine use. He felt that Coca-Cola purposely targeted children and didn't warn sufficiently about the caffeine issue. He saw that quite the opposite was happening: they were downplaying the issue and suggesting Coca-Cola was a harmless, fun beverage not associated with being a drug and the subsequent dangers.

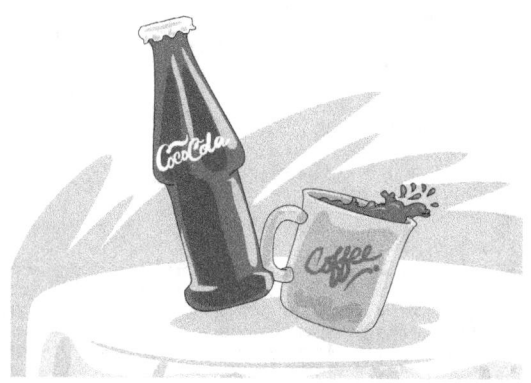

The Poison Squad

Dr, Wiley formed an all out posse, so to speak. He, along with twelve other volunteers, began to study the additives in such beverages. The fight between him and the leading soft drink company became an all out war. Dr. Wiley became famous by this point, and his campaign against the Coca-Cola Company was being observed by the entire nation.

He fought hard to pass pure food and drug legislation in regards to these issues. He felt strongly about these large companies' lack of responsibility on these issues, and for the sake of the children wasn't going to be bullied for standing up against them. Along with his "poison squad" he helped to create the first laws governing the caffeine content in beverages. The Pure Food and Drug Act was passed.

His first business at hand was to investigate the content of caffeine in the cola beverages; mainly Coca-Cola. The newspapers of the time were following this battle between the do good doctor and the largest cola company in the nation.

The company, led by John Cabdler, felt it was being bullied as well. They first had to fight long and hard to overcome the vicious rumors that the drink had cocaine in it. Then the caffeine content was being attacked. They also looked at how the nation embraced the use of coffee and tea and felt there was no way that cola should be singled out. It took many years for the company to overcome the cocaine rumors but it would prove to be a longer, harder battle over caffeine.

The Doctor vs. the Company

The two men at the forefront of the battle had many similarities. Each was well trained in the medical and chemical field. They had nothing in common though when it came to their view on this issue. Neither man had any issue with caffeine where it was a natural ingredient. The doctor however found that in cola this was an impurity element.

Some people saw the doctor as being far too strict with his chemical studies, but it was where his conscience led him. He saw the soft drinks as being extremely harmful to the younger generation, and he held this view until the day of his death.

Perhaps it was this strong feeling that motivated him to go overboard in his advocating for the use of coffee. He gave speeches on the subject as well as wrote many articles on the subject. While on one hand he was publicly speaking out against the Cocoa Cola Company, on the other he was praising coffee.

This inconsistency may have been the downfall for the doctor. In the end there was an obvious conclusion that most, including the federal government, came to. If he was correct in his estimation that caffeine was so harmful to children that cola should be banned, then it meant coffee and tea were also quite harmful.

Still the doctor insisted that parents were basically drugging their children each time they gave them cola. He proclaimed that parents lacked the knowledge they should have on the subject.

Cola vs. the United States

Eventually there would be a federal court case concerning the drug laws. This suit was between the government and the Cola industry. On one hand there were many religious leaders who made wild claims that the use of Coca Cola was cause for all kinds of debauchery in college dorms across the United States. They suggested that the use of cola led to sexual impurity and problems with insomnia. There were scientists called to support the claims of the religious.

The Coca-Cola Company also had its array of leading scientists who testified. They stated that claims being made were simply inconsistent with the known relationship between caffeine and human behavior.

One well-known and well-respected husband and wife team of professors did extensive studies on the subject. They did several thorough studies on the effects that caffeine had on the body. They concluded that in order to produce insomnia in an average adult, over 700 mg. had to be consumed. They also found that caffeine had positive effects like improving motor skills. These studies did little to address the real issues that Wiley had concerning the impact caffeine had on children. The Coca-Cola Company did, however, serve to discredit many of his claims.

In the end the Coca-Cola Company prevailed. It was ruled that caffeine was not legally an additive as it had been part of the original recipe. Another rumor was dispelled as the Coca-Cola Company acknowledged that in the original recipe trace doses of cocaine were included. Thus being that the drinks were properly labeled, there was no way the company could be found guilty of trying to deceive the public. They did voluntarily agree to stop targeting young children in their commercials.

The doctor lost one more battle with the company as he tried to have caffeine listed as a harmful addictive drug. He was quite famous from the court trial and thought the publicity might help him to get these provisions passed. In the end the cola company prevailed again and Wiley's suggestions were once more shot down.

Overruled

It didn't take long for the case to be appealed and taken before the Supreme Court. This time caffeine was ruled as an added ingredient. Also at time caffeine itself was on trial. The cola company settled the case out of court. Shortly after the settlement the amount of caffeine in Coca-Cola was greatly reduced. It is rumored that in so doing the federal government promised to leave the company alone from thence forth.

Coca-Cola Fights Back

A company as large as Coca-Cola doesn't become as large and important as it did by not protecting themselves from further such trials based on the federal government giving them their word. Recognizing the responsibility now placed on them, with caffeine being seen more as a drug than it had been, they formed "independent organizations" to help fight those trying to ban caffeine.

They looked at the history of the drug, much of what we have discussed in previous chapters of this book. They saw the potential for government or even religious fundamentalists to step in and try to regulate and forbid the use and sale of caffeine.

These independent organizations did many studies on the effects of caffeine and the human body. They publish these reports and they are scrutinized by other scientists who, by in large, find them to be credible. Of course we will never hear about any findings that would suggest caffeine isn't safe. We understand, due to their partnership with Coca-Cola, that they cannot be considered unbiased studies even if they are scientific in nature. Regardless of whatever loyalties they may have, the studies have helped many Americans come to understand a little bit more about the much consumed drug caffeine.

Cola Takes on the World

We mentioned earlier the main difference between coffee, tea, and cola being that cola is geared towards the younger generation. It is no secret that coffee and tea are, by in large, consumed by adults. So, in our health-conscious society it is quite surprising just how widespread the consumption of caffeine is amongst our youth. We often look at other countries that allow young children to drink alcohol and judge. Yet they are taught the effects and consequences from an early age, and the result is that there is less abuse in these countries than in countries that enforce age limits on the use of alcohol.

In contrast, here in America we don't enforce an age ban on caffeine but we also don't teach our youth properly about the effects.

Let us remember that when cola was first introduced it was sold like cold medicine in drug stores. When faced with how to promote their product, the large cola company decided to advertise its drink as a beverage that was safe for people of all ages. There were many within the company who would later come out and admit that they had great reservations about this choice made by the marketing team. They were well aware of the harmful effects that caffeine, if used in excess, could have on children.

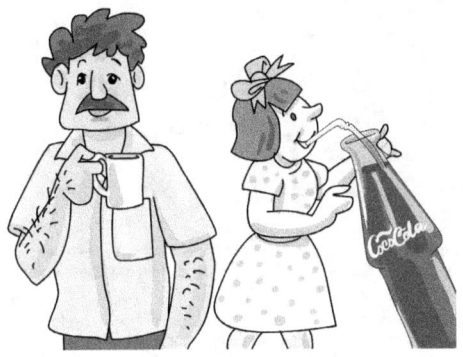

In the end money talks, and judging by the success of the company we can assume from a business standpoint they made the right decision. From an ethical standpoint one might cringe when we learn the history of Coca-Cola's public relations.

They worked long and hard at trying to entice the younger generation to become fans of their beverage, while still adhering to the promise they gave about not targeting very young children in their advertisements.

Jolt Sets the Bar Higher

The top selling soft drinks in our culture have always had caffeine in them. Following suit, other companies started to realize that the presence of caffeine meant the presence of cash flow when it came to the soda industry. Rather than be persuaded to decrease the dose of caffeine in their drinks, it was the beginning of a dramatic increase in caffeine for many products in the soft drink industry.

If you grew up in the 80s certainly you must have some memory of the soft drink Jolt. Jolt contained significantly higher amounts of caffeine than any of the soft drinks that came before it.

Jolt was proud to market its high caffeine content. The public relations team bragged that the drink contained twice the caffeine than other drinks. This campaign was in direct contrast to most soft drinks promoting a healthier image of their drinks. With twice the caffeine and twice the sugar you would think that the drink was met with widespread disapproval. On the contrary, Jolt quickly became well known and highly popular drink.

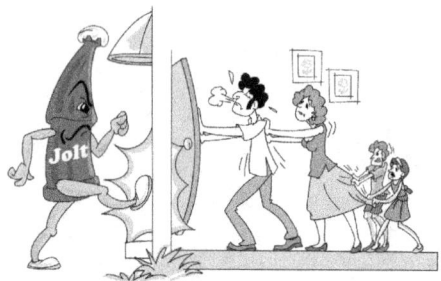

The drink was developed during the time that the coffeehouse revolution was taking place in American culture. University students, one more time, played a great role in the success of this highly caffeinated beverage.

In attempts to find a remedy to help them stay up all night studying for exams, students were seeking a solution that didn't include illegal drugs or legal ones rumored to cause heart problems and other medical conditions. Looking for something stronger than coffee but not as strong as illegal drugs, they found Jolt a good alternative. Jolt was like having a double espresso; however it had a less bitter taste thanks to the sugar content. It was also less expensive and more readily available, as it was sold in convenience stores and vending machines. Jolt was highly successful in its campaign to win over the college and university culture.

In some households children were strictly forbidden to drink Jolt, and there were stores that wouldn't sell it to anyone under the age of sixteen. The reason for this was widespread reports of hyperactivity in children after consuming the beverage.

In the 1990s many other companies soon came out with their own version of drinks like Jolt. Today Jolt is not sold in most stores as a result of so much competition. Yet there are still those who not only remember the drink but do their best to find it.

The highly caffeinated drinks have a certain bite in their taste. Many would argue that Jolt had a much more favorable taste in comparison to its rivals. The reason for the better taste had to do with the fact that most other colas used corn syrup and other sugar substitutes whereas Jolt uses cane sugar. There really is no comparison between the two components when it comes to taste.

Different Tastes

It depended on the flavor the company was going for in their caffeinated beverage as to whether or not the cola nut was used. While some drinks depended on different berries, others depended on the nut for the caffeine content it contained. It also had a distinct flavor that was sought after by some companies and avoided by others.

In South America there is a huge market for soft drinks. They use guarana in their drinks, and Coca-Cola has a huge investment in these drinks there. They mix the guarana with different fruits to create many different flavors.

The guarana-based drinks are hugely popular and the company cashes in on their popularity every day. Consider that billions of billions of quarts of soft drinks are sold there each year, and the guarana flavored drinks take up almost one fourth of the entire market.

The Pepsi Company has taken note of these profits in both Central and South America and has a marketing campaign targeted to introduce their own version of the drinks there.

By the end of the 20th century there were many new guarana-based drinks hitting the market in the United States. Some described guarana as a natural stimulant, but many disagree and claim that advertising the drug is irresponsible and misleading.

There was another drink that was introduced at this time called GUTS. This drink also contained guarana and had an even higher caffeine content than most others. The effects of the drink were quite noticeable, and it, like Jolt, became hugely popular amongst the younger generation.

The Day of the Energy Drink

Even with their high caffeine content, energy drinks still contained less caffeine than most coffee do. However, with the clever marketing of these new age drinks and the many fancy titles they hold, they seem to have a great appeal amongst the young.

One country seems to produce more energy drinks than any other. Austria is responsible for the creation of several of these highly caffeinated energy drinks. One of the most popular in the United States is Red Bull. Austrians consume extremely high amounts of the beverages and are responsible for much of the sales of the drinks in Europe.

In any industry that requires long hours late at night, doing somewhat mundane work, the popularity of highly-caffeinated energy drinks is huge. From computer programmers, to those working the night shift at the local gas station, you can almost guarantee an energy drink of some type is being consumed.

We can hardly talk about soft drinks that contain high amounts of caffeine without mentioning Mountain Dew. Early concerns about targeting the youth were well founded when you consider the popularity of drinks like Mountain Dew and Surge amongst the youth of today. They are responsible for billions of dollars in sales for the Pepsi and Coca-Cola companies.

There can be no denying when watching a commercial for these drinks that they target children. In fact, the companies do not deny that they intend to target the young male population. This makes sense when you consider that they purchase the most expensive advertisement slots running their new commercials during the Super Bowl and other sporting events.

Few people are aware that in some countries, due to the content of caffeine, Mountain Dew is considered illegal.

CHAPTER FIVE – FROM PLANT TO KITCHEN COUNTER

Let no man grumble when his friends fall off. As they will do like leaves at the first breeze. When your affairs come round, one way or t'other, Go to the coffee-house, & take another – Lord Byron - Don Juan

A Toxic Relationship

We know the effects of caffeine on the human body, but there is still much mystery in how plants developed the ability to produce caffeine in the first place. Caffeine provides a protective agent by the ability it has to destroy harmful bacteria and fungus. Caffeine also destroys any insects that would otherwise destroy the plant by causing them to be sterile. There is also evidence that caffeine has the ability to destroy harmful weeds that would strangle the plants if left to grow.

It seeps into the entire soil surplus and stunts the growth of the weeds. Caffeine's ability to kill harmful bacteria is only one of its amazing features in the plant world. Its ability to serve as an antifungal and insect killer could be a contributing factor in why the Coffea robusta plant produces a larger amount of the drug in comparison to its cousin plant: Coffia arabica. Coffia arabica is indigenous to Ethiopia and Yemen and doesn't require the same components for its survival.

The caffeine-bearing plants store and hoard the chemical components of caffeine throughout the plant body. They attempt to protect themselves by this action. However, in the end, because of the caffeine content in the soil around the plants, they ultimately are ravaged by the caffeine that once saved them. One way this happens is as the coffee plant grows they shed leaves and berries. The soil absorbs these waste products and becomes even more fertile with caffeine. The level of caffeine in the soil thus increases over time until ultimately it reaches a level that is deadly to the plant.

Coffee plantations can only survive as long as the soil stays above the toxic levels. The coffee plantation, after a certain period of time, will lose its profits rapidly as the plants are killed by the drug that helps them survive in the first place.

NASA Conducts a Study on Caffeine

A recent study on spiders conducted by NASA scientists suggests that caffeine can serve as a lethal toxin. This study used a multitude of different chemicals and showed how each affected the way the spiders spun their webs. Upon the influence of caffeine the spiders, like the mosquitoes in other studies, became disoriented and confused.

The theory is, the higher the toxicity level of the chemical introduced to the spider the more the web becomes abnormal. The structural component of the web allows for scientist to have the ability to cell by cell observe changes as they occur. Scientists use image data analysis to observe the changes in the web upon the introduction of the various chemicals.

They also observed spiders that were not under any type of chemical-induced stressed to analyze the images of the normal web. The study focused on the effect on the cells and the cell averages and radii of cells.

The NASA scientists felt that these studies, due to the cell structural component, could be done on humans and the findings would be the same. The results that they found are truly shocking. The reports of their findings were published in the biggest newspapers of our time.

What they discovered was that the caffeine proved to be toxic on many insects and it rendered the spider incapable of surviving. What wasn't reported in the much talked about findings was how caffeine performed as a defense system against the insects as a way of saving the plants.

They also didn't study the dosage given enough to truly make the comparison between spider and human consumption.

Bees and Caffeine

One insect that might have enjoyed the testing would be bees. They seem to be natural caffeine addicts. According to the story from a well-known beekeeper, he serves his yellow and black friends gallons of corn syrup every day. He suggests that bees seem to really enjoy the rush and they become extremely hyperactive. The beekeeper suggests that due to low levels of nectar, the bees naturally use the syrup and make a honey type substance.

It is no wonder the bees enjoyed themselves as the honey-like substance tastes a lot like the cola from which the syrup is taken.

The Coffee Shrub

There are many variations of the coffee shrub. The Coffea produces green leaves of a glossy nature and is a member of the madder family. It is responsible for a multitude of powerful pharmacological agents. Some agents composed from this variation of the coffee shrub include ipecac and caffeine.

There are several variations of the shrub that grow in tropical regions in the eastern part of the world. The appearance of the plant is often jasmine-like in nature. The comparison can be made between the intoxicating scent of the jasmine tree and the coffee shrub.

Coffee that we consume all comes from one variation of the shrub known as Eucoffea. The Eucoffea is the most economically important of the variations. There are still uses, though for the other variations. They are used as stimulants and décor, however the fruit shouldn't be eaten as it may cause severe stomach cramping and other medical problems.

One species known to be indigenous to Ethiopia is said to be the first cultivated species. It is called Coffea arabica. Today it is found mainly in Latin America and is represents the majority of coffee consumption around the world.

Another highly sought after species can be found in Africa and other countries. This is another species that is economically important. Mainly cultivated in Asia, Coffea roubusta is said to have originated somewhere near the Congo.

The third species found in Liberia is said to create a strong intoxicating blend that is much higher in caffeine than the coffee we are used to. It has a larger and sturdier chemical makeup than either the Coffea arabica or Coffea robusta versions.

In addition to the others we add coffea *excelssa*, which was discovered in the early 20th century. The beans, much like the Coffea liberica, are high in caffeine and much sturdier than the others.

Coffea arabica was introduced to Brazil in the 18th century. That country quickly became the largest coffee exporter in the world.

Theobromine vs. Caffeine

Cacao is popular for the way it stimulates users. The agent responsible for enhancing this effect is the theobromine component. Cacao powder generally contains a much higher dose of theobromine than caffeine. The levels of theobromine found in the cacao beans varies dependent upon the type of plant. The levels can also be affected by the fermentation process.

Theobromine is taken out of the seed husk and is much less potent cell by cell than that of than caffeine. High levels of theobromine can work as a diuretic. Theobromine, if taken in the proper dose, can also serve as a muscle relaxer and heart stimulus. Theobromine can serve as an agent initiating vasodilatation.

A study conducted in the late 20th century at a prominent medical university found some interesting answers as to which agent was responsible for the effects. In the study, caffeine was given to different subjects at graduating doses. Then the same subjects were given theobromine in the same graduating degrees.

It was discovered that the subjects had a much higher threshold for theobromine than they did for caffeine. The caffeine was found to be significantly more potent. Dose by dose this seemed to hold true amongst all subjects. There is much more theobromine found in chocolate than caffeine. The higher levels of theobromine present in chocolate make it hard to determine exactly which chemical is more predominate.

A glass of hot cocoa, compared with a glass of chocolate milk, has about ten times as much theobromine than caffeine. The average candy bar was shown to bypass the threshold for theobromine in approximately twenty percent of the subjects, while caffeine produced a much higher percentage rate of subjects exceeding the threshold.

The universal findings showed that caffeine likely has a much more powerful stimulating effect on the average person. However the effects of both theobromine and caffeine on the subjects were similar. The duration of caffeine's effect was much shorter but began quicker when compared to theobromine. There also seems to be proof that caffeine affects the body in more dramatically than theobromine.

The Mate Plants

One of the top five sources of caffeine that is imported and exported in the world is yerba mate. The drink most associated with yerba mate is called *Gon gouha* which refers to the plant that it was infused from. Gon gouha is the most consumed caffeinated beverage in South America. It also serves as the way that most South Americans get caffeine in their diet.

The most popular mate comes from wild trees. Several hundred thousand tons of yerba mate leaves are cultivated each year, containing three thousand tons of caffeine. A notable percentage of the entire world's supply comes from this cultivation. It is estimated that billions of cups of mate are consumed each year in South America alone. There is also a huge exportation of the plants and products that come from the mate of Brazil to other South American countries.

Mate Drinks

One plant that grows in South America is a species of holly said to grow up to nearly one hundred feet tall. The leaves are large and dark, growing over half a foot in length. The holly plant produces flowers that form near the end of the branches. It takes between two to six years before the plant can be harvested. The plant reaches it peek at ten years and levels out at twenty years.

A popular beverage made from the holly leaves begins with the harvesting of the unopened leaves of this plant. Due to the height of the plant, the process of getting to these leaves can be quite dangerous. The natives must clear away vines to get to the leafiest branches.

In order to maintain the harvest, the largest branches are left untouched. The branches that are cut are taken to a factory to be processed. The entire process takes several hours, and great measures are taken to ensure that the caffeine content is not lost in the process. It takes nearly eighteen months before the leaves are finally processed and ready to be turned into the popular South American tea.

Some of the natives are said to have used yerba mate for its stimulant effects and as an agent to fend off disease. In parts of South America, mate drinking is a way of life, much like coffee drinking is in the West. The people spend many hours consuming the beverage. It is easily the most popular caffeinated drink in that part of the world. One writer in the 1800s found that mate was most like tea, but that it wasn't nearly as good and shouldn't be considered an equal substitute. Another writer also compared mate to tea and hinted that despite what the scientist say he felt that mate didn't pack the same punch as tea did.

There have been many studies done on the properties of mate. The level of caffeine in the drink ranges between one to two percent. The less mature leaves have higher levels of caffeine. Mate can also be prepared in a variety of ways. These properties make it hard to determine accurate levels of caffeine in the drink itself. It is suspected that theobromine can be found in mate, although that has yet to be properly detected. The inability to detect theobromine suggests that if it is present the dose would be too small to produce any effect.

Well before the 1500s, the natives of South America were using mate to make beverages. Much the same as coffee and cocoa in other lands, mate was used as a means of trade to the natives.

The leaves of yerba mate can be infused and consumed. They use a reed which serves as a straw to drink from the calabash in which the drink is created. A strainer is used to get out sediment, much like the process of brewing coffee.

There are many different names for the plant. Some natives called it "caa," while the Spanish are said to have called "Yerba". It was welcomed with open arms by those occupying the colonies and they found it very enjoyable.

In some countries, during the middle of the 16th century, religious leaders took over the areas where the plants were being grown and began cultivating for themselves. This may be why the drink received another name "Jesuit Tea" which it is still called to this day.

The beverage is prepared mainly the same way that tea is. Water is boiled and then poured over the leaves. However the gourd is then passed around. When the tea-like beverage is prepared in the traditional South American manner, boiling water is poured over the dried leaves in a small silver-mounted calabash about the size of an apple. In family circles the beverage and a straw-like apparatus are passed around like a tobacco pipe in Native American circles. It is more often found today though that it is served in cups with straws.

Each cup uses an ounce or two of the leaves. People often use different sweeteners to add flavor to the drink. Due to the ability to use the same leaf over and over again, it is hard to estimate the exact content of caffeine in the beverage. It is estimated that the drink can be most easily compared to a weak cup of coffee.

Today, mate leaves can be found in stores selling health foods or homeopathic remedies. They are used in several different types of tea as well. One interesting fact is that products containing mate are often labeled as caffeine-free when in fact that is not the case.

North American Drinks

There is another holly plant referred to as "cassina," which is found in the Appalachian regions of North America. The plant has been used for hundreds of years to make a hot, stimulating drink with the same name. In the sixteenth century, early explorers described a drink that was used in ceremonies. They said the drink was black and used as a medicine. One captain of that time found North America to be a place that was suitable for the French. Upon relocating to North America they were given many cassina plants. The plants were also used for trade purposes.

There are Native Americans in the 20th century that are reported to have used the plant for its medicinal purposes. They fast and stay up for several days using the plant as a means to do so.

Chemists in North America began curing the plant. One product of the curing process resulted in a beverage known as cassina mate, which resembled yerba mate. However despite the best efforts in the U.S. to promote the drink none was ever successful. The failure is probably due in nature to the similarity of the drinks and tea. Most would agree tea tasted better and was more effective.

The Guarana Plant

The guarana plant is native to the Amazon. It has fruit that is small in nature and usually has only a single seed. It has very large leaves and flowers that grow in clusters. The guarana seeds were named after the Guaranis Indians.

The seeds are roasted like the coffee bean, and once done brewing a very popular drink is created. The drink is popular in South America for its stimulating effects. The drink is said to even smell like coffee but it is more bitter in taste. The seeds, however, have a much higher caffeine content that the coffee bean. During the 1800s the guarana was used as medicine because of the high caffeine content. The yoco tree is a sister to the guarana, and yoco bark is used to create a caffeinated beverage.

Guarana seeds are made into a fine powder through a series of steps. The powder is then mixed with water and put into containers. Then, once they are the right texture and color, many different products can be made.

This is the process used to make tea as well as guarana bread and cocoa. The beans are mixed in hot water along with a sweetener to prepare the tea for serving. This tea has a much higher caffeine content than coffee. The tannin process of guarana and yoco also create a foamy lather which is used in some countries as soap. However when used in lakes and streams the saponin as it is called seems to render the fish confused.

Some believe that the beverage is a panacea and they carry sticks to grate the plant. The natives use fermented crushed seeds infused with hot water to create a less than pleasant smelling drink.

Today, guarana has become popular as a carbonated drink with similar effects of cola. The United States has seen its share of guarana-based drinks grow in the twenty-first century. It is often an ingredient in teas as well. Guarana powder is sold as a new organic product, which is obviously just another misleading advertising move as it has been around for centuries.

Guarana pills are even sold by advertisers who exaggerate the history of guarana. They boast about guarana's ability to work as a sexual stimulus in men.

It was in the 1600s that guarana came to be known by the Western World. It was in the 20th century that companies started to really campaign to commercialize guarana. It has become one of the most sought after tonic plants in some South American countries. In the United States guarana use is spreading, especially among the health conscious.

CHAPTER SIX – THE NON-CAFFEINE COMPETITION

"Ah! How sweet coffee tastes! Lovelier than a thousand kisses, sweeter than muscatel wine! I must have my coffee . . . Johann Sebastian Bach

Other Natural Stimulants

There are other natural alkaloid stimulants besides caffeine that are used to create a great diversity of beverages. Below we will discuss some of those stimulants that compete with caffeine as natural uppers. We will also discuss the sources from which they come.

The Coca Plant

Native to the Andes Mountains, the coca plant is a small tree with tiny white flowers. It is the source for the powerful addictive drug known as cocaine. The leaves of the coca plant have been used a stimulant dating back to ancient times. The natives chewed on the leaves for energy while working at high altitudes and to suppress appetite when food was scarce. The leaves can also be mixed with lime for the same effect.

Typically it takes close to twelve months for the seedlings to be ready to leave a nursery. The cultivation time, once the seedlings are replanted, depends on many variants. One variant is where the seedlings have been relocated too. Another factor is how big or small of a plantation they have been relocated to.

During the spring and fall, if the plants are the proper size (approximately five to seven feet in height), they are harvested. The leaves are gathered and then cured. Once this process is complete they are dried and powdered. When the process is complete the leaves can be sold for their intended purpose.

The demand for coca around the world outgrew the supply in South America and other countries stepped in to meet the demands. This resulted in the East Indies becoming the leader in the legal trade of coca to nations around the world.

Powdered coca leaves are sold at local markets in the countries native to the plant. As a means of working long hours on little or no sleep, the local laborers chew the leaves for sustenance.

There are areas where distance is determined by how far one can get on a single chew of the leaf. Generally, to produce the desired effect, the leaves are mixed with lime, which extracts the alkaloid known as cocaine.

The use of the coca leaf itself doesn't seem to have any real negative effects on the society where the natives of the land chew it regularly. The consequence of using the extracted cocaine are however often devastating on societies where it is consumed. Cocaine use often results in dependence. The person dependent on cocaine suffers with episodes of rage and paranoia. Cocaine dependency can lead to permanent psychosis.

The Effects of Extracted Cocaine Use vs. Chewing the Coca Leaf

It is still unclear why there is such a dramatic difference in the effects that chewing the coca leaf has on a person compared with the use of the extracted cocaine.

The rate of absorption when chewing the leaves is considerably slower than that of someone smoking or injecting it. It is also suspected that perhaps other alkaloids can only be activated when smoked or injected. It would make sense then why simply chewing the leaves gives the much less dramatic effect.

It is not as easy as it may sound for scientists to discover the reason for the considerably different effects. Scientists have many of the answers but still lack the ability to say exactly why these psychoactive plants do what they do.

Khat: the Tree and the Drink

In a late 19th century book written about tea, there is mention of an Arabian tea called "Cathadules." The tea is created from the leaves of a shrub that is said to be grown and cultivated solely for the purpose of creating the tea.

The tea is as popular among the natives as coffee. The tea is also referred to in some text as "Abyssinian tea." Like the coca leaves, the leaves of the shrub are said to be very intoxicating.

The Khat tree - also referred to by many other names such as; qat, kat, chat, and miraa - is a shrub-like tree whose leaves, when fresh, are chewed for a stimulating effect. The twigs can be chewed as well. The popular drink made from the Khat tree goes by the same name and is popular throughout the Eastern World. In Yemen, the country that it is traditionally known as the home of coffee, khat has been part of the social network for many years. Like coffee, khat is used in both vocational and residential settings. Khat is a popular beverage consumed by the masses. In other close by countries the drink is much less popular. It is mainly used only by those with professions that require long nights with no sleep, and is not used regularly by most of society.

The Europeans were introduced to khat after its popularity in the Eastern World became known to them. Many believe khat is equal in potency to tea and coffee. This being the case, most people just assumed that khat contained caffeine. Scientists have discovered, however, that khat doesn't contain any caffeine; it contains alkaloid stimulants that structurally resemble amphetamines. The active ingredient, cathine, is responsible for the effects of khat. Another attribute of the cathine and norephedrene is the effect it has on the brachial tubes. Many reports suggest that there is an enlargement of the brachial tubes.

Studies on khat conclude that the leaves hold much more cathine than either cathinone or nor ephedrine. They also show that after they have dried, the khat leaves lose most of their potency. The use of khat had not spread like the use of the coca leaves. One reason that khat is much less popular is the bitter taste it leaves on the pallet after being chewed. This, along with it being much less potent, makes for little competition between coca and khat.

In the Middle East khat leaves are chewed and then they form small balls that people pocket in the side of the cheek. This makes for a lasting effect throughout the day.

In the 21st century, reports show that bundles of the khat branches sell from anywhere to under a dollar to over forty dollars depending upon the quality of the branch. To acquire enough khat to really feel the effects costs the average person in the region about half a week's wages.

The men of the Yemen gather together in their homes and chew the branches and leaves; sometimes this can be an all day event. Many people chew khat during their work day and others who, for one reason or another, need to be awake all night.

Unlike other countries, the leaders in this region openly embrace khat and use it themselves as well as require a supply for military men. Their use of the plant has been documented by journalists covering civil unrest in the region.

In Yemen, the country that it is traditionally known as the home of coffee, khat has become popular among the men. Khat use is becoming popular amongst the females in society as well. They have parties of their own, like an English tea party, with khat being the main focus of the gatherings. They serve other beverages to combat the cotton mouth that results from khat use.

Those Opposed to Khat

Certain scientists and professors have spoken out against the use of khat. They suggest that regular use of khat can cause gum disease, loss of appetite, and impotency. The scientists believe that the feeling of well-being that goes along with the use of the plant only encourages its users to become hooked on seeking out that feeling that only khat can give them.

Ironically the reports that some scientists and professors put forth to warn against the use of khat note the very same effects that others who extol its virtues. There is also the social aspect to its use. Like coffee and tea, khat gatherings bring people together who otherwise would not interact. In an area where neighboring tribes are often at war, this aspect is especially positive in the eyes of those in power.

Those promoting its use also swear that the plant is not addictive, and they look to the fact that most people don't travel outside of the region with the plant as proof of its non-addictive nature.

In Yemen, over three quarters of the land is used in the cultivation of khat along with an equal portion of the water supply. This is one reason some in government there are trying to reduce the use and production of khat. Thus far any measure taken to prohibit its use has fallen short.

Ephedra

Ephedras bear small cones and are a relative of the pine tree. They are native to many regions of the world and there are several different genuses that contain the drug ephedrine. Ephedrine is a stimulant alkaloid whose main pharmacological use is in the treatment of asthma.

The stems of one species are said to create a bitter but stimulating tea. The dry stems are boiled with hot water, and this practice has been done for centuries in some countries.

The Mormon settlers in the United States were rumored to have made a tea from ephedra and they felt it was acceptable to drink as it wasn't a caffeinated beverage. Caffeine was strictly forbidden in the Mormon religion.

The Chinese made a highly potent medicine from three different species of the Ephedra tree. They have used this combination for centuries. The use of ephedrine was common there long before they knew anything about tea. The alkaloid extracted from certain species of the trees has been used in the West to treat nasal and bronchial conditions as well as treating heart and lung problems.

Today, the synthetic versions of ephedrine are more often used as herbal stimulants and are sold in pharmacies or health food stores.

The FDA has recognized a tendency among the young to use the ephedra products as appetite suppressants and for its stimulant quality. The abuse of ephedra can lead to many health problems including death, especially in young users who take far more than is recommended. The young users often combine the use of ephedra with caffeine which adds to the danger.

There are many ways the plants can be used. Once harvested they are dried out and then cut into pieces. If it is to be used as a medicinal powder it is first boiled and then roasted.

Many countries still use ephedra to treat diseases and colds. It is also used to treat pain. Cold medications and many allergy medications, both prescription and nonprescription, contain synthetic ephedrine or pseudonorephedrine.

Ephedrine is also used among certain populations for its speed-like qualities. Truck drivers or those in other occupations needing to stay up all hours of the night use ephedrine. Ephedrine is often sold at convenience stores and truck stops for this very reason.

Betel

The betel pepper and the areca palm are both referred to as "Betel". They go by other names as well, such as the pan plant or the betel palm. The seed of the areca palm along with the leaf are used as a stimulant in many eastern countries. They are chewed together to produce the desired effect. A large portion of the population has a regular habit for chewing the betel. It can be compared to chewing tobacco in the Western World.

Introduced in the fourth century, the palm was first cultivated in the Western Indies. The tree can grow to be anywhere from twenty to fifty feet tall. The radius of the trunk is only about a foot though. The palms reach up from the top. Before the fruit of the tree has a chance to ripen it is picked then boiled and laid to dry in the sun until it tans. Generally the fruit is about the size of a large egg.

It is the alkaloid arecoline in the betel nut that acts as the stimulating agent. It can be used as a worming agent in animals. The wood of the tree can be used for dyeing and tanning and is known as the "black catechu".

Natives in the East have used the betel palm for thousands of years. In the 1300s the Chinese were said to have been chewing betel. For more than two thousand years the natives of the regions where the "betel palm" grows have used this drug. One famous explorer, Marco Polo, traveling in the 1300 and 1400s gave detailed reports of how he encountered a people continually chewing on the betel palm, often mixing it with other nuts and lime.

The reports suggest that the natives were addicted to chewing the plant. They were said to have enjoyed the plant so much that they paid no mind to the habit of simply spitting out one bunch of leaves in exchange for the next.

Marco Polo was surprised to find that even among the royals this habit was extremely popular as it was said to be an extremely healthy habit. The royals were also in the habit of mixing the leaves with other spices to add to the flavor.

One writing in the 17th century described betel and lime chewing. He included it on a list of other heavier drugs such as opium and less potent one like coffee. It was said to be used by people of all ages and classes. There was no discrimination in the religious circles either, they all used betel. Entire population of the time seemed to be addicted to the betel.

Preparing the Betel

The betel is often prepared by combining it with the nut of the areca palm. It is mixed with a fresh leaf and flavored with lime, pepper, and other spices that enhance the bitter taste. Users add spices that aid in bringing out the active alkaloids by increasing salivation. The saliva actually turns a burgundy color from chewing on the leaves and it colors the lips and gums. Some claim that it also stains the teeth but this seems to be inaccurate according to recent studies. Scientists figure that the rumor got started since many in the regions where the betel is popular have poor hygiene and most likely had black teeth before ever chewing on the leaves. Also there are certain tribes who use other means to dye their teeth as it is seen as a sign of beauty and health.

Yohimbe

Yohimbine is a crystalline alkaloid that comes from the bark of an African tree. It is the bark that is referred to as yohimbe. It is said to have a spicy flavor, and also spices up the love life of its users. The Africans have claimed for years that the yohimbe is a natural aphrodisiac.

In the Western World it is used in teas and occasionally marketed as an aphrodisiac. It is not that common in the West as scientists haven't done enough testing on the drug. They suggest that the reason it is said to increase ones sexual appetite is because it actually acts as an irritant to the urinary tract. It works much the same way that cantharides do in livestock.

Some scientists claim that it has no aphrodisiac powers at all, but that people taking it for that purpose are most likely already sexually stimulated and wrongly attribute that to use of the plant. Researchers think there may be unknown chemicals in the bark, but yohimbine by itself wouldn't produce the effects it is said to be responsible for.

The active ingredient yohimbine acts as an antagonist to the auto receptors. This affects the body's thermostat and adrenergic activity, which in turn affects the temperature of the body as well as the brain's ability to recognize temperature changes. It results in a decrease of noradrenalin production. This causes the body to reduce the amount of heat it produces if the temperature outside the body rises.

They are unlike other auto receptors in this way in that they amplify the noradrenergic activity, which is the main reason they can be used to treat impotency. Scientists have long known that increased adrenergic activity is said to stimulate sexual function.

It is also used to treat anxiety and other heart-related conditions that lend themselves to an increase of adrenergic activity. However it is very important that Yohimbine never be combined with any other stimulants or MAO inhibitors that are commonly found in many prescription drugs. This combination can be lethal, so users of yohimbine must exert extra caution when combining the plant with any other drugs.

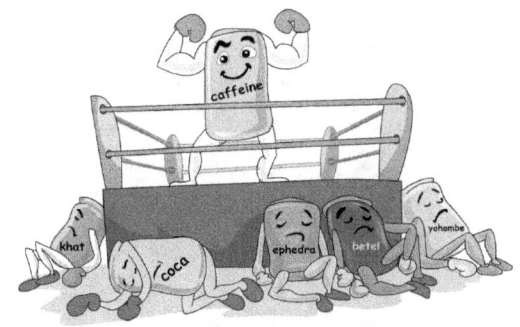

Caffeine and Tea: the New Partnership

Celestial Seasonings, one of the most popular tea makers during the 20th century, began to embrace caffeine in its once famed non-caffeinated teas. They only had a handful of teas with caffeine in them but those few accounted for over eighty percent of the tea sales.

The company began to market their tea and advocated for users to really become aware of caffeine and how it affects the body. They showed on each box what the caffeine content was in relation to that of other popular caffeinated beverages including coffee, cola, and chocolate. It created awareness that coffee wasn't the only means of getting caffeine for that morning or afternoon pick me up.

The Coffee Addicts' Coffee

Spike is the Jolt of the coffee world. It claims to contain almost double the amount of caffeine than that of a regular cup of coffee. Spike markets its beverage to those who consume coffee purely for the effect. Much like Jolt, they brag about the high caffeine content and repeatedly reference it in their advertisements. They actually show people injecting coffee in their veins in their ads.

The beans used to produce Spike are generally robusta which are much less expensive than the Arabica variety. This is of little concern to Spike drinkers though who are not drinking Spike for its taste but for its caffeine content.

Caffeinated Water

In the l990s, with the introduction of so many caffeinated beverages, it seemed almost natural that "Water Joe" joined the scene. This beverage was artesian well water laced with caffeine. It bragged about having no artificial flavors or calories. The marketing team didn't suggest you skip your morning cup of coffee but that you add their beverage to your morning for an extra added energy boost.

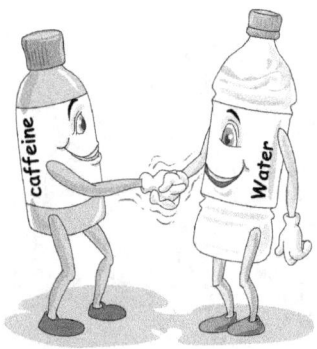

Two groups heavily targeted by the marketing team were athletes and health conscience people. These groups didn't want to drink coffee as it was thought to cause dehydration if not properly balanced with water intake. The bigger market was the large amount of people who really don't like the way coffee tastes but do enjoy the energy boost they get from drinking it.

The creator of the beverage was among this group of individuals. He looked back at his University days and recalled a strong dislike for colas and other caffeinated beverages like coffee and tea. He noted that his classmates though who were frequently drinking coffee and other beverages had an extra boost that he was missing and desperately needed for studying.

The company claimed that the drink tasted just like pure water but contained as much caffeine as a cup of coffee. There is no label to tell exactly how much caffeine it contains. It is true that it doesn't contain calories or sugar, or any added preservatives.

Can it really be all that and taste like water? The jury is still out on that one. In tastes tests people are fairly split in their opinion on that subject. Although even when the caffeine taste was detected it was barely noticed.

Caffeine and Alcohol

Starbucks, in their marketing genius, partnered with a brewery and created a malt beer that was targeted at both coffee and beer drinkers. The man in charge of the brewery company says the idea was conceived during a conversation over coffee. There was much testing and mixing of flavors to come up with the final product.

Neither company wanted to lose their flavor. The brewing company naturally wanted the beer taste to be noticeable, while Starbucks wanted the coffee taste to predominate. There was an incredible synergy amongst the two companies and the end result was a product that both were extremely happy with and proud of.

Simply put, they added coffee to the beer and the result was miraculous. Starbucks chose a combination of Arabica beans and Central American coffees which gave the brew the strong aroma of coffee with the rich full taste of a stout. They called the drink the "Double Black Stout."

Pepsi and Starbucks Join Forces

Pepsi-Cola joined forces with North American Coffee Partnership during the same time period and created a product that was essentially a carbonated coffee. It is sold at Starbucks as well as in other stores. The drink is supposedly a new version of a drink that was used by the foreign militaries more than one hundred years ago.

PepsiCo also created a drink around the same time that was another carbonated coffee beverage but with a cola flavor added to it. They marketed this combination of coffee and cola as the best of both worlds.

Turbo Cake

Not to be left out, Coca-Cola came up with a product that was a mixture of Coke and espresso, which they called Turbo Cake.

Marijuana and the Coffee shop

Amsterdam, where marijuana is legal, never bothered with the attempts that other countries did at banning caffeinated products. They have a long history of tolerance, and the coffee shops there are places where people can openly purchase and smoke marijuana.

People from around the world travel to these area coffee shops where they can enjoy a nice cup along with smoking a joint or two. Leaders encourage the youth to use the coffee shops as it is a safer place for them than they might otherwise find. There is funding from the government to support these coffee shops. Unlike in other countries where it is illegal and frowned upon, there isn't as much of a problem in Holland with addiction and crime associated with marijuana.

A Change Underway

In recent years people have found tea more and more enjoyable. There are many different types of specialty teas and this has created a great enthusiasm for them. Some would say that the popularity of tea is rivaling that of coffee. Others would argue that's simply not the case.

In the major North West cities, best known for coffee, they have seen a dramatic increase in the amount of people drinking tea.

It is not just in the United States but in other countries where teahouses are beginning to open again and they are becoming quite popular in places that were traditionally dominated by coffeehouses.

There is much speculation as to why this sudden increase in tea drinkers. One reason may be the social attributes of tea drinker versus the coffee drinker. Tea again is seen as the more sophisticated beverage.

For some people it is a matter of taste. There are many people who simply don't enjoy the taste of coffee. With all the flavored teas now available it makes sense that this segment of society would be swayed to drink the flavored tea. There are even micro brewed teas. Tea shops are opening in all the same places as coffee shops. Many universities now have both. There are tea bars in grocery stores and colleges, including the most prestigious colleges in the United States.

One sign that tea time might be here for the long haul is that Starbucks now sells a variety of different teas.

Caffeine Use to Reduce Caffeine Use?

Many people that have been misinformed about caffeine. There are those who take advantage of this in order to promote their own alternative caffeine products. They are always promising equal or more powerful benefits. Ironically, in most cases, one of the main ingredients in these products is, in fact, caffeine or caffeine compounds that we known to be very dangerous if mixed with ephedrine. One of many ads promoting one such product claimed that due to its guarana base it helped people by reducing the craving for caffeine. The same product contained caffeine as one of the active ingredients. Many of these products that come out claim to be "new" panaceas; but if you do just the littlest of research it is almost certain that of the two active ingredients caffeine is one.

Guarana

Guarana is said to have been used for centuries for energy and alertness. Guarana plays an important role in Tupi and Guarani Brazilian cultures. The plant was introduced into Western Civilization during the 1600s. Guarana is rich in caffeine and is said to have nearly triple the caffeine content than coffee has. It is used in some popular cola beverages, and its drinkers enjoy the energy and stimulation it is said to give them. Guarana, like coffee, is said to suppress the appetite and even relieve the symptoms of PMS along with headaches.

Caffeine Pills

There is an increase in awareness of the benefits of using caffeine-based pills over drinking coffee. There is no need to always be in proximity to coffee stores or restaurants. There is no need to determine just how much caffeine you're getting in a specific cup size, or finding out what type of beans are being use. Pills also cost less and it is much easier to control the dosage. . Further, there is no cholinergic acid in the pills and there is some research that the acid inhibits some of caffeine's benefits.

Some manufactures and distributors combine other stimulants with the caffeine to create a dangerous mix. There is only one company that sells a pure caffeine tablet. Thermo Power Boost® combines pure caffeine with EGCG (a derivative of green tea) the provides the fat-burning capability of the caffeine without increasing the caffeine content. In fact, a 100 mg. tablet of Thermo Power Boost® provides the fat burning capability of 500 mg. of caffeine!

Some manufactures make wild claims about their products. Thermo Power Boost® caffeine tablets improve one's mood, fight off fatigue, and improve physical performance.

They didn't claim, as some others before them have, that caffeine could dramatically enhance physical and mental abilities. They also didn't suggest that the pills would increase memory or endurance.

They made sure to include a warning that caffeine should never be a substitute for sleep. They cautioned users to learn how caffeine affects them before increasing the use of the product, as the effects can vary from individual to individual.

Any tablet or pill that contains one hundred milligrams or more of caffeine must contain the following warning: "The recommended dose of this product contains about as much caffeine as a cup of coffee. Limit the use of caffeine-containing medications, food, or beverages while taking this product because too much caffeine may cause nervousness, irritability, sleeplessness and occasionally rapid heartbeat."

Due to a lack of federally accepted studies on the matter, they cannot claim that the pills boost physical and mental coordination. They can't claim how the pills help people memorize facts. They are limited to stating that caffeine can improve the mood, boost confidence, and increase alertness.

They stick to the status quo and suggest the pills may help boost the mood for bodybuilders as well as reduce mental fatigue. They have good reason to stay within the confines of safe and federally approved claims and they make sure to do so.

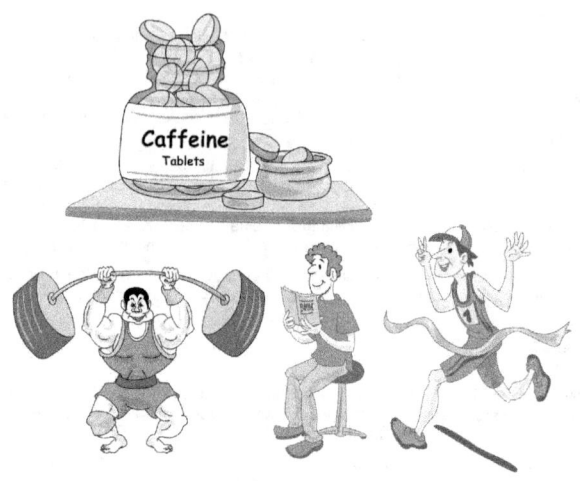

CHAPTER SEVEN – CAFFEINE . . . AND THOSE WHO USE IT

The morning cup of coffee has an exhilaration about it which the cheering influence of the afternoon or evening cup of tea cannot be expected to reproduce. ~Oliver Wendell Holmes

Studies done to look at patterns of caffeine consumption have been few and far between. There has also been only limited research into the patterns of how people use caffeine and how often they use it. In the United States, a few such studies have been conducted, while elsewhere the research on this subject has been even more limited.

The following patterns have been observed in some of the studies that have been done on this subject:

1) People use caffeine more as they age. Once they are between forty to fifty years of age they tend to stop increasing the amount of caffeine they consume. As the approach old age (post sixty five) they tend to slightly reduce the amount. The fact that people tend to increase the amount of caffeine as they age confuses studies on the long term healthy effects.

2) There seems to be no difference in caffeine consumption between males and females. Women and men metabolize caffeine differently, and this along with considerable weight differences make studies in this area a bit skewed as well.

3) Over eighty-five percent of the individuals asked in the study admitted to using tea and coffee. When cola drink and other foods that have caffeine in them is also a part of the diet, caffeine use approaches 100%. One study showed only a minimal percentage of the country didn't use any caffeine at all.

4) A study done in other countries found that over ninety percent of the population used caffeine on a daily basis. Based on these figures it is estimated that worldwide over ninety percent of the population uses caffeine on a daily basis. This leaves between three to eight percent of the population as occasional users.

5) The view on what beverages are the most popular or the most out of favor changes with time. One professor at a leading University concludes that when it comes to alcohol, the attitude changes approximately every seventy years. Many people don't realize this pattern because it only changes once in their lifetime. In the United States, for example, alcohol consumption peaked towards beginning of the 80s and has been on a gradual decline ever since. You can note this decline most in the sale of distilled spirits.

When it comes to coffee, it just makes sense that it will follow the same type of cyclic patterns. In the last hundred years the use of caffeine has increased dramatically worldwide. This pattern is seen in specialty coffees as well as regular coffee.

On average, most adults in the United States consume between two hundred to three hundred milligrams of caffeine a day. The higher range is from those who admit to being caffeine consumers. According to some standards this would mean a huge portion of the population falls into the area of being caffeine dependent.

In countries outside the United States consumption rates of coffee are much higher. Some countries brag that they consume three times as much coffee as people in the United States. There are at least ten other countries that rank as larger consumers than the United States. One of the top is Finland with its population consuming more than double of what Americans do.

During a twenty year period, from the 1960s to the 1980s, the United States saw an almost forty percent drop in coffee consumption. One study done during the same time period showed that a large number of people simply quit drinking coffee altogether.

The study done during these years showed that while coffee use was on the decline, soft drink consumption was on the increase. The highest selling soft drinks all contained caffeine. This being so, the overall caffeine intake didn't decline much as people just switched from coffee to soft drinks.

Caffeine: the Drug of choice for Baby Boomers

A well known article that was one of the first to do a survey of the baby boomers found some interesting facts. This study was conducted in the 1990s on baby boomers who were born in the 1940s. The results showed a majority of people were happy with their sex lives, unhappy with their chosen professions, and nearly one fourth admitted to being hooked on caffeine.

It was interesting to note that this generation, so well known for their use of recreational drugs, listed caffeine as their drug of choice. One reason for this was that nearing middle age many of the "flower child" generation had grown up. Still seeking a stimulant of some kind, many of the baby boomers found coffee to be the perfect solution. There is no question that coffee wasn't being served at Woodstock or other wild drug parties in the 1960s. With the heavy use of drugs like methamphetamines, Acid, LSD and heroin it is not surprising that it wasn't until many years later that the baby boomers would even notice coffee.

It may have taken that many years for the baby boomers to become aware of the dangers of both illegal and pharmaceutical drugs. Once clear on that they were sought a safer high that increases alertness without being dangerous to the mind and body. Caffeine has proven to be the answer. As long as used in reasonable quantities, caffeine poses no danger whatsoever to its users.

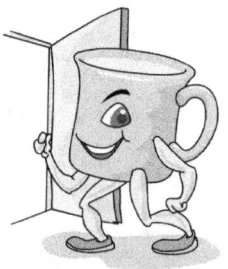
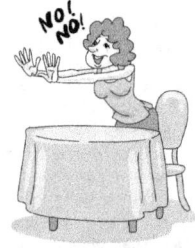

Coffee and the Next Generation

There may still be some prejudice against those who hang out in coffee shops. There are many who see the coffeehouse as a place where idle chatter goes on and people sit around doing nothing for sport. Coffee holds the image of being a drink for those over the age of twenty-one, but this image seems to be becoming more and more inaccurate.

In the 21st century, coffeehouses are the regular hangout for teenagers, and even pre-teens. These youngsters are consuming coffee and other caffeinated beverages at the same pace as those much older.

Why would the young generation want to hang out in the same establishments as the businessmen and older members of society? For one thing, the hours that coffeehouses are open is just perfect for kids either on their way to school or coming home. They can meet there in the early morning before school and hang out. Perhaps they are looking for that image of sophistication that they see drinking coffee will give them.

There is an obvious bonus with the coffee shop as well. They serve minors: no ID checks at the local coffee shop. Children are allowed to get high legally. What could be better for a teenager? Most parents would rather have their children hanging out at a coffee shop than on the streets or in malls.

A Safe Alternative

With so many things off limits for children it is no wonder that they are turning to coffee shops and the use of caffeine as a way of crossing that long bridge between adolescence and adulthood.

Naturally there are people who are worried about this and question what the long term consequences to these trends will be.

There is no evidence thus far to suggest that caffeine is harmful to children if consumed in a reasonable quantity. Also, considering the alternatives, what parent would really object to having their teenage son or daughter drinking coffee here and there?

There is one last reason that some teenagers may turn to coffee. Consider the number of teenagers in the 21st century that are addicted to alcohol and drugs. There are hundreds of treatment centers nationwide that are for teenagers alone. Once these kids are out of whatever rehabilitation program they were in, they are usually encouraged to go to twelve step meetings, and at every meeting nearly everyone is drinking coffee. Thus coffee becomes a much safer drink of choice for many of these youngsters recovering from other deadly addictions.

CHAPTER 8 - CAFFEINE: THE PSYCHOLOGICAL & PHYSIOLOGICAL EFFECTS

Conscience keeps more people awake than coffee. ~Author Unknown

Caffeine into the bloodstream and beyond

Caffeine absorbs into the bloodstream rapidly through the intestines and stomach. Caffeine is water soluble and quickly enters all cell membranes. Caffeine is then carried and distributed to the organs of the body. It doesn't take long after consumption for caffeine to be present in every cells of the body.

The body doesn't contain any organisms that serve as a barrier to caffeine's entrance in the blood stream. Caffeine is distributed more evenly than other drugs. Studies conducted on caffeine, and how it affects the body, show that the concentration of caffeine in different bodily fluids is very close to being equal in each. Some of the fluids that were tested included; breast milk, blood, and saliva, which all proved to hold an equal amount of caffeine.

Caffeine's ability to serve as a stimulant is enhanced greatly by its ability to quickly enter the central nervous system. It must be able to cross the blood-brain barrier. It has to get beyond the mechanisms that serve as a defense for the central nervous system. The central nervous system is protected from toxic exposure by only allowing smaller molecules to enter the brain or the spinal fluids. This mechanism blocks out viruses from attacking the body. The body is able to withstand certain drugs even when they are injected, because of these defenses. For reasons not fully understood, caffeine has the ability to cross these barriers with ease.

Coffee reaches its maximum exposure threshold in the body approximately sixty minutes after being consumed. The stimulating effects are, by then, felt throughout the entire body, including the brain.

In soft drinks, it takes a bit longer for caffeine to be absorbed. In both beverages the absorption rate is dependent on the person's weight. One person weighing one hundred pounds would feel double the effects as that of another weighing two hundred pounds.

The Human Body and Caffeine Absorption

There are a number of dynamics that affect the way the human body absorbs caffeine. Factors that slow metabolism include: pregnancy, oral contraceptives, liver damage, genetics, and alcohol. Some of the factors that speed metabolism include: cigarette smoking, age, and body size. These different factors account for how many people give different reports on how caffeine affects them.

The Liver's Role in Caffeine Absorption

The liver is responsible for purifying almost all chemicals ingested by the body. Caffeine travels via the bloodstream to the intestines and the stomach then throughout the body via the large vein that runs through the liver.

The liver converts the caffeine into metabolites, which are then flushed from the body during urination. Almost one hundred percent of the caffeine consumed is excreted through the body in this manner. The small percentage that remains doesn't change.

It is a complicated transformation that caffeine undergoes, and there are more than a dozen metabolites produced during the process. Studies vary greatly due to different rates of metabolism in subjects. Experiments done on rodents demonstrate different rates than that of monkeys for example. Thus, any studies done on animals are really of little help in better understanding how caffeine affects humans, as the absorption rates are considerably different in animals than in humans.

We've already mentioned the body's ability to absorb caffeine rapidly and quickly eliminate it from the body. The reason for this is that caffeine has a high solubility in water. Caffeine doesn't remain in the organs of the body due to how rapidly it passes through the tissue. Also aiding in this is the fact that caffeine is not fat soluble and therefore cannot sustain in the body's fat storages. If it could remain in the fat reserves it would be retained for considerably longer periods of time. Other drugs remain in the body's fat storages areas for many months.

The Half-Life of Caffeine

Half-life is a term that scientists use to refer to the amount of time it takes the human body to rid itself of half of the amount of chemicals ingested. The half life for caffeine is approximately four hours, and in less than twenty-four hours over eighty-five percent of the drug is entirely absent from the body.

This elimination process can be affected again by the many variables we've discussed earlier. An example would be the rate at which a pregnant woman and a non-pregnant woman metabolize caffeine can differ by almost twenty percent. Pregnancy dramatically increases the half life of caffeine. Newborn infants metabolize caffeine at much slower rates than adults. The most logical explanation for this dramatic difference is the liver's important role in metabolizing caffeine. The newborns liver is incapable of producing the necessary enzymes, and thus caffeine stays in their bodies for many days.

The use of other drugs also affects the metabolism of caffeine. Smoking increases the rate, while drinking alcohol slowers it. This means that drinking alcohol with your caffeine assures you will feel the effects much sooner. Smoking has the opposite effect. With both of these drugs it has much to do with the way they affect the elimination rate of caffeine.

A Closer Look at Smoking and Coffee Drinking

Coffee drinking and smoking have been linked together since the beginning of the coffeehouse. Many in the writing profession are known to be heavy smokers and coffee drinkers. Most of the first coffeehouses were also known for the cloud of smoke in which one was enveloped as he visited with his fellows.

As we look at the way smoking affects the body's ability to metabolize coffee it helps us to understand why the two seem to go hand in hand. It even helps us to see why coffeehouse owners would encourage their patrons to smoke. A smoker has to drink nearly double the amount of coffee than that of a non-smoker to achieve the same desired effects.

We can also understand better why attempts at using caffeine to help in the cure and prevention of alcoholism have occurred. Caffeine cannot change the amount of alcohol in the blood but it can alter the mental impairment that one feels when intoxicated. Caffeine is felt more by a person who has been consuming alcohol and thus the stimulating effect is more profound in that person than it would be in a sober person.

These studies prove that there are many variables at play when it comes to just how caffeine affects a person. It is important to understand that not all medical doctors understand or embrace these scientific findings.

We would never suggest you ignore your doctor's advice when it comes to the use of any substance. We only encourage you to consider the many variables at play when it comes to any decisions you make about caffeine.

That Thing You Do

Even those opposed to caffeine recognize its ability to increase energy, improve clarity, and enhance alertness in most people. As a means of understanding why caffeine is able to affect people in this manner, and just how it does so, has been studied more than any other drugs.

Since their introductions, tea and coffee have left scientists and chemists wondering just exactly how do they do what they do? One scientist in the late 1800s believed that the body had a desire to store xanthine, which is known to be found in small doses in the body's tissues. He suggested that caffeine naturally satisfied this desire because the structure of the two was so similar. Scientists today have dismissed his theory but do acknowledge that caffeine is indeed a member of the xanthine family.

Caffeine produces more than one effect on the central nervous system as well as other organs of the body. This makes understanding the drug complicated at best. This complex nature has made it impossible for scientists to all agree on caffeine's mechanism of action. The biggest mystery is how caffeine acts as a psycho-stimulant and the way in which it affects the cardiovascular system.

How Other Stimulants Work

In looking at the ways other drugs affect the body we may be able to better understand the way caffeine works. Mainly we will look at stimulants such as cocaine and amphetamines.

All stimulants act as either agonists or antagonists in the body. Agonists stimulate a response, while antagonists inhibit a response. Agonists are able to stimulate a response by the way in which they affect hormones and neurotransmitters. This affects the rate in which nerve cells fire.

Antagonists inhibit the action of a drug, also through neurotransmitters, causing them to fire less energetically. Had they been allowed to reach their uptake sites, drugs would caused the nerve cells to fire more or less frequently or energetically. Essentially the agonist creates more of a charge, while the antagonist lessens the energy present. Amphetamine and methamphetamine work as agonists. Methamphetamine enters the brain and triggers the release of norepinephrine, dopamine, and serotonin. In high concentrations it acts as a monoamine oxidase inhibitor, stimulating the mesombolic reward pathway, which results in the feeling of euphoria and excitement. Withdrawal is characterized by excessive sleeping, eating, and anxiety.

Cocaine works as an antagonist. Cocaine inhibits the uptake of dopamine. This results in higher levels of dopamine being present in the synapses. Many of the same feelings are experienced by cocaine users as the methamphetamine users.

It is more often in the agonist groups that dependence occurs. Drugs in this group are more prone to produce tolerance requiring users to ingest more of the drug for the same effect, thus resulting eventually in a growing dependence.

Drugs in the antagonist category don't tend to require users to use more of the substance. A person can take relatively the same amount and achieve the same effect. They certainly are known to be psychologically addictive but they are not physically addictive as tolerance is never achieved.

We discussed earlier that caffeine is indeed the most studied drug, and it may also be the least understood. Science of course has advanced and the studies being done today are much more conclusive than those of the past; however they are still very much debate on many matters. Modern investigations into the pharmacology of caffeine are both intricate and inconclusive. Results are simply hard for even scientists to interpret and rely upon.

In the last twenty years there have been at least three widely accepted theories. The three are: Calcium Mobility Theory, Phosphodiesterase Inhibition Theory, and Adenosine Blockade Theory.

The calcium mobility theory is no longer considered viable because the average person would have to drink approximately one hundred cups of coffee before this could happen. That makes this theory relatively meaningless when it comes to understanding how caffeine affects the body.

For the same reasons, the phosphodiesterase Inhibition theory is not used because the average person would have to consume between forty to fifty cups of coffee in under ten minutes to get the results described in the theory.

The adenosine blockade theory is now the accepted standard. Caffeine is known to work as a pain killer and mood enhancer. It also can serve as a means of suppressing the appetite. Caffeine can do these things by the way it regulates the neurotransmitters. A neurotransmitter can only perform the function it is designed to perform if it can successfully reach its destination in the central nervous system. There are substances that block the neurotransmitters from reaching their destination and thus render them ineffective.

One such drug is called adenosine: used to treat a variety of conditions. Some side effects include decreased urination. Serving as an inhibitor to the nerve cells, it affects the way other neurotransmitters respond, especially the ones affecting excitability and responsiveness.

This theory suggests that caffeine acts as an antagonist of adenosine, blocking the uptake and effects of adenosine. The result from this blockage is that caffeine prevents the body from the depressing and hypnotic effects of adenosine. This theory first surfaced in the 70s and explained why caffeine keeps us awake when we should be tired. It also accounts for caffeine's ability to increase respiration and the frequency of urination.

There are, like the other theories, many variables to consider. Adenosine receptors vary and have many roles in the cell structure and tissue.

Caffeine plays a role in the pharmacology of adenosine; it is just hard to determine to what degree. Alertness is affected by the neurotransmitter's ability to function in the noradrenalin system. In people who use caffeine chronically, changes can occur in the neurotransmitters that affect the level of norepinephrine, dopamine, serotonin, acetylcholine, GABA, and the glutamate systems in the brain.

Only much more extensive research can provide conclusive answers to how caffeine use really affects these changes. Recent findings show adenosine may well relate to caffeine's action as a stimulant and link it to the same behavior in other stimulants, including cocaine.

Other research suggests that caffeine enhances dopaminergic activity, as it serves as an antagonist to adenosine. If this research is correct, then caffeine produces behavioral effects at the dopamine receptors and, like the other well known stimulants, it would mean it produces increased synaptic concentrations of dopamine. There are more and more studies that suggest this may be a true action of caffeine.

More Questions than Answers

Any regular coffee drinker knows that in time you build a tolerance to coffee, and most would admit to at least some form of dependence on it as well. Thus lies one of the major problems with trying to label coffee as an antagonist or inhibitor. A major paradox arises when we attempt to understand caffeine's primary effects in terms of its role as an adenosine antagonist, or reuptake inhibitor.

There are obvious symptoms to withdrawing from caffeine. This can be said of any beverage or substance that contains caffeine. Over time a person builds up tolerance, and if consumed on a regular basis, the tendency for dependence of some degree is likely to happen. This has been established in many scientific studies and documented throughout history in literature.

Speculation has arisen due to the way in which caffeine seems to produce an increased amount of brain adenosine receptors. Scientists believe the body is fooled by caffeine's role as impostor, and thus creates new receptor sites in an attempt to compensate. If caffeine intake is reduced, then the extra sites merge with the others and uptake a greater amount of adenosine. The result is that sleepiness and depression, which caffeine was counteracting, are now intensified. This could explain the withdrawal symptoms caffeine users face when they quit.

Some Inconsistencies

Certain questions arise that make scientists wonder if the evidence is complete. Again, the explanation for caffeine tolerance isn't fully explained. When a person uses caffeine long enough they can reach a point where no matter how much caffeine they ingest they will not feel the effects. This inability to surmount the tolerance threshold is inconsistent with the adenosine blockade theory.

Another problem is the lack of a competitive antagonist likely losing its potency after being repeatedly used. Caffeine doesn't follow this pattern; it retains its full level of potency even if up against an insurmountable tolerance. If caffeine's role as a mechanism of action worked as a competitive blockade of adenosine, you would expect to see symptoms of withdrawal upon cessation of use.

Problems like this help us to understand that there is still much work to be done when it comes to fully understanding how caffeine affects the human body. We are able to study the effects of caffeine on the body in other ways that don't rely on fully understanding all of its underlying mechanisms.

Where the Caffeine is

Most people in the United States have never gotten their caffeine from chewing the parts of plant that hold caffeine. It is through soft drinks, tea, coffee, chocolate and other foods and drugs that we get our fill of caffeine and caffeine-like compounds. The following is a breakdown of where most Americans get their caffeine:

Source	Percentage
Coffee Beans	65-70%
Tea Leaves	12-15%
Crystal Caffeine	13-14%
Cacao Beans	2-3%
Other Natural Sources	2-3%

We know that theobromine is responsible for most of the stimulating power found in chocolate. Theophylline is responsible for some of the same effects found in tea. There is an added extract in cola drinks that accounts for the caffeine found in them.

We also know that there are many over-the-counter, non-prescription and prescription drugs in which caffeine can be found. Drugs used for alertness or even pain killers contain caffeine.

One study found evidence linking high blood pressure to coffee consumption. The study was conducted over a forty years on a group of medical students. Once they were able to rule out all other variables, the link between drinking coffee and the hypertension seemed to be quite apparent. Of course there are other scientists who say that there are still too many variables to reach this conclusion, and even the scientists who did the research tend to agree with that analysis.

Another study was done over a much shorter period of time, but on a larger group of people, took people who already had high blood pressure and then subjected them to regular consumption of caffeine from different beverages all containing caffeine. The study found that the caffeine use had virtually no affect on the high blood pressure. The conclusion was that caffeine didn't cause hypertension.

There have been a multitude of studies done on this issue, and most research suggests that those who have hypertension should proceed cautiously when it comes to using caffeine. Some studies have found an increase in blood pressure, heart rate, and work load on the heart after taking caffeine. In those study, some who already had hypertension seemed to show a marked progression when they began to regularly consume caffeine. The results among people who didn't have a previous condition varied, and only one person showed any notable change towards the onset of hypertension after the caffeine consumption.

Once the study concluded, the end result was that it was suggested for those with hypertension to avoid using caffeine when exerting themselves physically. There are millions of people who suffer from high blood pressure. This is probably the most dangerous effect caffeine could have on one's health. The jury is still out on how caffeine affects the unborn fetus as well the new born infant. Though some research suggests that pregnant women should not use caffeine as there has been a link to caffeine use and miscarriage. Yet, a new study showed that moderate coffee drinking by overweight pregnant women led to more normal birth weight babies with more ideal metabolisms.

The Effects of Coffee vs. Caffeine

Coffee doesn't seem to affect the intestines in the same way as caffeine. Caffeine stimulates the small intestine to release sodium and water but coffee doesn't appear to do so. Coffee does stimulate the colon, and people often have a bowel movement after drinking coffee, but research has shown it most likely is another agent in coffee responsible for this effect. People drinking non-caffeinated coffee have the same response.

Another study showed that in both decaffeinated and caffeinated coffee there was an increase in the levels of gastric acid after consumption (this is less true for organic coffee). They also had an effect on the esophageal-sphincter tone. Scientists don't yet know which agent in coffee is responsible for these effects.

Caffeine seems to upset the stomach and cause an increase in acid which can cause pain in existing ulcers, but there has been no evidence that caffeine is the actual cause of the development of the ulcers themselves. Once again, it doesn't seem to be the caffeine in coffee that can account for these aggravations in existing ulcers. There is enough evidence to suggest that coffee either causes or at least aggravates heartburn in certain individuals. When coffee is added to water it causes more reflux than caffeine. These findings all suggest another agent at work.

Impossible Variables

Some studies on the human body are difficult to conduct. There are so many variables at play in individuals it is often hard to really know if a study is objective. Part of the way scientists can take facts from hypothesis in research is by being able to conduct the study over and over and get the same results. With humans this is nearly impossible.

Also there are obvious limits on what human beings can be exposed to. Adding to the complication is the role of the brain on how thought may impact subjects. Specifically, when it comes to studies done on caffeine's effects on the body, one problem is that the group of people who are selected may all be from the same region or race making it a biased sample group. Another potential problem is that the exposure a person has to caffeine is often hard to measure. The person could be getting more caffeine in their diet than they are aware of. This brings us to the last problem which encompasses them all, which is the impossibility of excluding all variables in human subjects. There are obvious things that can be done to prevent animals from certain variables that can't be done with humans.

One place we see the obvious nature of this dilemma is in the study of how caffeine affects the human fetus, both before and after birth. Scientists are trying to determine if caffeine can affect any of the following: delay conception, miscarriage, low birth-weight.

The majority of studies couldn't determine a correlation between caffeine use and these conditions. It is also important to understand that even the people conducting the tests are subject to bias, whether intentional or not.

Most books on pregnancy to date advise women to limit or avoid caffeine use. But some of these conclusions are based on incorrect samples being taken in these studies due to a lack of understanding on reproductive hazards when caffeine is the primary focus.

Exposure

In order for research on caffeine to be accurate, you must be able to measure the exact amount of exposure to caffeine. We already discussed that, due to many different variables, this can be quite difficult. In trying to understand a dose relationship it is important that those conducting the studies don't increase levels to get the sought after results.

Often times research shows low exposures being correlated with low risk, moderate exposure with moderate risk, and high exposure with high risk. This can lead to scientists being more likely to expect these results and disregard evidence that suggests otherwise.

In conclusion

We have discussed the way in which variables can influence the results of studies conducted on caffeine and caffeine's metabolites on human health. Many scientists feel that it is these variables that are responsible for many inaccurate reports when it comes determining the effect of caffeine on pregnancy.

We can look at the mother's age as another variable, and as we know caffeine use increases until middle age, when most women are beyond child bearing years. Thus arises another variable. Other risks occur in women when it comes to pregnancy and age that have nothing to do with how much caffeine they are consuming.

CHAPTER NINE – CAFFEINE: THE HEALTH BENEFITS AND DANGERS

Caffeine isn't a drug, it's a vitamin! ~Author Unknown

Caffeine: The Scapegoat

It seems that society often sees those things we deem pleasurable as being bad for you. We look at things like stimulants and, despite contrary evidence, we blame all types of behaviors and conditions on them. This is especially true with caffeine and coffee. They have both been looked at with suspicion since their introduction. No matter how many reports come out stating that caffeine poses no real health threat there will be those saying otherwise.

Coffee and caffeine are said to be the cause of many degenerative and malignant diseases. While there is no proof caffeine causes any of the following here is a list of some diseases often linked to caffeine:

1) Hypertension/High Blood Pressure
2) Cancer
3) Anxiety
4) Heart Attack
5) Osteoporosis
6) Gout
7) Insomnia

Before caffeine was known to be in coffee, tea, and chocolate, those substances were linked to curing or causing many conditions. On one hand they were hailed with being able to positively influence physical and mental health. On the other hand it was suggested they caused anxiety, insomnia, etc. Most people to this day are confused by all the conflicting evidence that comes out about caffeine.

Caffeine and Depression

There were early reports from travelers in the East that caffeine was a healthy drug that takes away sadness, subdues anger, and generates cheerfulness. One writing in the 17th century on depression had an epigraph later added discussing the use of coffee and its ability to cure melancholy.

The doctors of that time (1600-1800) were respected, and once they gave their approval of caffeine it seemed its popularity quickly spread. In an early advertisement for a caffeinated beverage there was a list of conditions that caffeine was said to cure.

The list contained many diseases and conditions that the common man was suffering from during the 17th century.

It was suggested that if a person, especially an elderly person, experiences melancholy early in the day all they need is about two cups of coffee and they should feel a boost in both their physical and mental condition.

Caffeine and ADD

A recent debate that has emerged is whether caffeine use is linked to attention deficit disorder. Evidence suggests that caffeine can induce the symptoms of attention deficit disorder, but it is also used as a cure. There are other studies "proving" caffeine has no affect whatsoever on the condition. This is the perfect case to show the complex and confusing answers that one is faced with in trying to determine whether caffeine is good or should be avoided.

PMS: worse with caffeine?

Almost fifty percent of females experience some lever of premenstrual syndrome one to two weeks before they begin their menstrual period. There are over one hundred symptoms said to be linked to premenstrual symptom, and these can be debilitating for some women. Some of the most common are; irritability, tiredness, breast swelling and tenderness, headache, anxiety, depression, cravings for chocolate, acne, and changes in sleep patterns. For some women these symptoms only last a few days, for others it can last the entire two week period. As a woman ages the symptoms become more severe. Scientists haven't yet determined exactly what causes the condition but many women seek anything that will help them combat the symptoms.

There have been studies that claim caffeine aggravates the symptoms of premenstrual syndrome. One study conducted on almost one thousand women was attempting to find a link between diet and premenstrual syndrome. The study included all varieties of caffeine intake. The results were that women who consumed caffeine were much more likely to suffer from premenstrual syndrome. When the caffeine was consumed, an assessment of caffeine intake from all sources was made. Even drinking just one cup doubled a woman's chances of suffering from the syndrome. They compared different doses and found that the more caffeine was consumed, the more women suffer.

Some physicians claim that caffeine increases the likelihood of symptoms like insomnia, anxiety and irritability. They suggest that reducing caffeine intake provides quick and immediate relief. It has been suggested by some doctors to reduce or eliminate caffeine in the diet before the cycle begins.

The jury is out as to whether or not caffeine indeed makes the symptoms of premenstrual syndrome worse or not. There have been many studies that would suggest it does. Even cutting caffeine out entirely will not result in all symptoms of PMS disappearing.

Caffeine and the Risk of Osteoporosis

When a woman suffers from osteoporosis it often results in pain of the neck and back along with changes in posture and loss of bone tissue. Bone tissue is made up of calcium. Naturally anything that decreases a woman's calcium uptake or secretion needs to be avoided, especially in post menopausal women who are much more likely to develop osteoporosis. The relationship between caffeine and calcium is complex. Some research suggests that it creates an increase in the amount of calcium that is eliminated from the body; however it doesn't appear to affect the body's ability to absorb calcium.

A study done on pre-menopausal females, and the relationship between caffeine intake and the risk of osteoporosis, concluded that caffeine didn't pose significant risk to women. The study suggested that women use caffeine moderately, and only if they are healthy with normal or increased amounts of calcium in their diet.

A more recent study looked at the intake of coffee over the span of an entire lifetime and how it affected bone density in the spine and hip. Over nine hundred women participated in the study. They used X-rays to study the bone density throughout the years of coffee consumption.

The results were very convincing that coffee reduced the bone density in the spine and hip. All other variables were considered and ruled out as the cause for the reduction in bone density. The study also showed that if women drank milk it could counteract the effect that coffee had on bone density, but calcium supplements couldn't.

Yet another study looked at the relation between caffeinated cola beverages and osteoporosis. The results indicated that women who consumed caffeinated cola beverages had significantly lower bone mass density at the hip, but not the spine. They found no similar association in men. They also found no association with the bone mass density loss and the consumption of other types of non-caffeinated sodas.

Caffeine and Pregnancy

We assume that pregnant women exposed to higher doses of caffeine are subject to higher risk, and studies conducted often come to this biased conclusion.

Using a control study along with placebos is important when doing this type of research. Scientists often use decaffeinated coffee as a type of placebo and as a way of knowing the exact dosage of caffeine

The average cup of tea or coffee contains between six to fourteen ounces. This is a variable that needs to be determined when discussing the affects of one "cup" of coffee on a person. Also, consider that each coffee bean can produce different amounts of caffeine. The manners in which the beans are brewed also affect the caffeine content.

Another factor is that answers test subjects give on questionnaires are often found to be unreliable. Many people answer quickly and either over-estimate or under-estimate their caffeine consumption. One study on a particular type of cancer found that the reported amount of caffeine ingested and the actual amount found varied considerably. Some underestimated the amount of caffeine they consumed and others over estimated the amount.

When it comes to studies on pregnancy, women are more likely to underestimate the amount of caffeine. In women who had suffered a miscarriage they seemed to report a more honest amount of caffeine consumed.

It would seem there is much room for error in any study trying to understand the metabolites of caffeine. There are problems again with answers to questionnaires, as well as problems with the ability to rule out all the variables we've discussed when it comes to caffeine exposure.

Since the body changes so much throughout pregnancy, it is difficult at best to measure the exposure to caffeine. In pregnancy there are even more variables at play, including the speed of metabolism and how it changes throughout the period. When women are feeling nauseated they are less likely to consume caffeine. Also, consider weight gain in pregnancy and how that affects the action of the metabolites on the body.

For reasons unknown, near the end of the third trimester the body rids itself of the metabolites at a slower rate than in the first trimester. This creates in some women unpleasant feelings and therefore women reduce the amount of caffeine they ingest.

There is another problem when focusing solely on the effects of caffeine: scientists overlook other drugs that may be the cause of certain effects. There are many medications that include caffeine as we know, and often these medications are not looked at when these studies are preformed.

Caffeine and Age

As a person ages, caffeine begins to affect them differently, and it is important to be aware of this change. People, generally speaking, consume more coffee as they age until reaching midlife where they usually stop increasing the amount. The way that caffeine affects them changes over time as well.

There has been much research on how caffeine affects people at different stages of life. One study looked at how caffeine affects the psychomotor performance of people as they age. In the younger and older age groups, caffeine seemed to enhance performance. In the older subjects the improvement was seen in attention and reaction time, whereas in the younger subjects the improvement was in motor speed. Overall, this study showed that caffeine had more of an impact on the older subjects than it had on the younger.

Caffeine and Sleep in the Elderly

Once people reach middle age they tend to lose an average of one to two hours of sleep a night. What most people, young and old, don't realize is that many prescription medications contain caffeine and contribute to sleeplessness. Even over-the-counter drugs used to treat headaches or minor aches and pains contain caffeine.

One study of at least two thousand people past middle age showed that a significant number of them were using medicines that contained caffeine. Many people in that same group reported troubles with sleep. The study showed that due to the fact that many people are unaware of caffeine being in other products, they tend to consume them in the evening, and those products affect their sleep.

The study also showed that certain juices can increase the amount of caffeine in the bloodstream and greatly affect any medications a person may be taking.

People who often suffer from having cold feet and hands may have other more serious conditions that are causing that. It is especially common for older people to experience this. It can be caused by circulation problems and should always be brought to a doctor's attention to rule out anything serious. It could mean that people with this condition should avoid caffeine, depending on the root cause.

We've discussed in other chapters how certain cultures claim caffeine works as an aphrodisiac. There has been a recent study done in the United States that suggest this is the case, especially amongst the elderly. The study found that senior citizens who were regular coffee drinkers tended to be more sexually active than those who were not.

Vision and Caffeine

Caffeine is known to constrict blood vessels. This may affect a person's vision and also increase the risk of contracting glaucoma. Caffeine can't cause glaucoma, but for people who are already at risk of developing the disease the use of caffeine can increase the risk.

A different study came to the same conclusion, deducing that in people who already had the disease caffeine intake made it worse. But amongst those who were healthy there seemed to be no effect on the pressure to the part of the eye that is susceptible to glaucoma. The rate at which the caffeine was consumed also seemed to play a role.

Like other drugs that work as a stimulant, caffeine dilates the eyes and can affect a person's ability to focus. Cocaine and amphetamines have this same affect, making it difficult, especially at short range, to see clearly.

Caffeine and Nutrients

A study conducted on animals and caffeine showed that caffeine negatively affects the body's ability to store important nutrients like calcium, magnesium, and zinc. The scientists believe that the response seen in animals could be similar in humans. Another study showed that consuming caffeine before a meal affects how much iron is absorbed. Iron deficiency has been shown in studies to be closely linked to caffeine use.

Caffeine in the Therapeutic Community

There has been a recent increase in studies focused on caffeine pharmacology and how it is used to treat peoples' conditions. The main focus has been on how caffeine can be used as a diuretic and a cardiac muscle stimulant. It has also shown promise in elevating plasma levels and relaxing muscles. .

Caffeine and Headaches

We already know that caffeine has been used for many years in both prescription and non-prescription pain killers. There is conflicting research on the actual benefits of caffeine in this area. Some studies suggest that the presence of caffeine in these drugs makes them almost doubly as effective. It doesn't mean it will kill more pain, only that you have to take less to kill the same amount of pain.

People have used caffeine to treat headaches due to the way in which caffeine acts as an antagonist, and how it affects the blood vessels on the cerebral cortex. Caffeine affects vasodilatation: a contributing factor for severe headaches.

Caffeine can also enhance the action of ergotamine, which is also used in the treatment of migraines. People suffering from migraines found that coffee and certain alkaloids together brought much relief. It is thought that the relief comes from caffeine's ability to increase ergotamine's oral and rectal absorption in the body.

Autonomic Failure and Caffeine

There have been studies done to see just how caffeine affects people with low blood pressure. Low blood pressure is caused by autonomic failure. People often become extremely weak and can faint when they stand up. The body doesn't respond to the need for a rise in blood pressure while doing things like eating or standing up. The body's organs, such as the lungs, heart, and intestines, are all affected by this loss of motor function in the nervous system. In one study, people were given around two hundred milligrams of caffeine to combat the condition. It seemed that the subjects needed to refrain from consuming caffeine for a period of time beforehand to really get the sought after effect. Doctors suggested that drinking one to two cups of coffee in the morning can help people with autonomic failure.

Caffeine: Improving Skin Conditions

Caffeine, in cream form, has been used to treat many different skin conditions. There are several different conditions that researchers have studied using caffeine including pruritus, erythema, scaling, lichenification, oozing, and dermatitis. Caffeine is able to extract water from the skin tissues and this may be part of how it works in helping combat the conditions listed above.

One form of eczema most often found in children and new born can cause tremendous physical pain. The condition known as atopic dermatitis can even become debilitating in some patients, especially those who suffer with it in adulthood. Caffeine has shown to significantly reduce the symptoms of the condition.

There are products for those with normal healthy skin using caffeine as well. They are now being used to treat wrinkles and to firm the skin.

A recent study showed amazing results in caffeine's ability to prevent and treat skin cancer. This study found that in animal studies, cancerous tumors were reduced almost seventy five percent, and caffeine was nearly forty fiver percent effective on non cancerous tumors.

Caffeine and Parkinson's Disease

A recent study conducted on over seven thousand men showed that high consumption of caffeine can lower the risk and slow progression of Parkinson's disease. The study was conducted over three decades and it found that the men who drank more coffee had less incidence of Parkinson's than those who only drank a little. It also showed that the men who drank even the smaller doses had fewer incidences of the symptoms than the men who drank no coffee. The study showed the same results from other caffeinated sources as well. They believed caffeine was affecting the motor symptoms.

Another scientist found similar results and credited caffeine's ability to block adenosine receptors resulting in higher levels of dopamine. People with Parkinson's suffer from lower doses of dopamine so it would make sense that a drug which increases dopamine levels would be effective as a treatment.

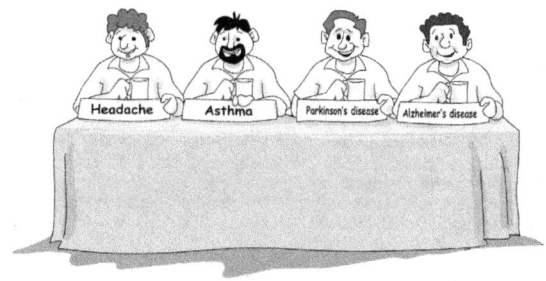

Both doctors agree that even though the results seemed to be conclusive, there must be more research done before they can be certain about caffeine's ability to help in the prevention and treatment of Parkinson's. Though the outlook is very promising from studies conducted so far.

Caffeine and Cholesterol

Studies conducted on several thousand people, both male and female, find there seems to be no relationship to caffeine and death in these high risk groups. Earlier studies done suggested there was a relationship between people with high blood pressure and high cholesterol and the use of caffeine. It was noted caffeine use in these groups could result in serious health complications.

It is very important to understand that where coffee is ruled out as having no relationship to certain diseases it means caffeine is ruled out as well. However if coffee is said to show a link to a certain disease it doesn't necessarily mean that caffeine is part of the equation. As we discussed already coffee has many metabolites and characteristics that caffeine doesn't have. It could easily be these other agents that are the cause for whatever link there may be with coffee and disease.

Caffeine and Blood Pressure

Despite early reports that suggested otherwise, in regards to blood pressure, coffee can actually help lower it. The cardiovascular effects of caffeine are no secret. Almost every study conducted over a long period of time reveals evidence that suggests caffeine can actually prevent certain types of cardiovascular damage.

Unfiltered coffee contains particles that can raise the risk of cholesterol and pose danger to the cardiovascular system. It appears that long term consumption non-filtered of raises the cholesterol, but filtered does not. This is one case where coffee is linked to these conditions but caffeine is not.

One such study was conducted on more than ten thousand men and women with high blood pressure. The researchers found that women who consumed more than six cups of coffee were at no more risk than those who didn't consume any. The same was true for an even larger scale study done on men that showed no link between coffee, caffeine, and cardiovascular disease.

These results confirm what other findings conducted over the past twenty years suggested, which is that coffee has "no influence on the rate of coronary heart disease." They also showed no evidence that supports the hypothesis that higher levels of caffeine consumption are related to death rates from strokes in hypertensive patients.

Another study conducted over a thirty year period came to the same conclusions: that there was no direct relationship between caffeine intake and elevated blood pressure except in the first few days of use; before the body builds up a tolerance.

So when it comes to answering the question, "does caffeine have any effect on blood pressure?" it would seem to be that it only affects blood pressure in the first few days of use, and that this effect quickly disappears. This initial exposure is the only time caffeine seems raise a person's blood pressure.

After all the debate over whether or not coffee raises blood pressure it is quite interesting to note that some studies suggest coffee can actually lower it. Studies done on this subject suggest that if used on a regular basis, coffee can, in fact, lower blood pressure. It showed that for every two cups of coffee consumed, patients showed a one point decrease in diastolic and systolic pressure.

The study showed that people who drank coffee on a regular basis seemed to overwhelmingly have lower blood pressure than those who didn't.

There were studies done that showed there was no association between caffeine consumption and death among hypertensive as had once been suggested. We already know that when you consume caffeine it will raise blood pressure slightly for the first few days. This actually means that it may be better for those with hypertension to drink small amounts of caffeine daily than to only drink it occasionally.

There is even evidence suggesting that the use of small amounts of caffeine daily may reduce the risk of developing high blood pressure in high-risk groups. A study showed that people in the high risk group consuming at least a cup of coffee a day actually had lower blood pressure than others who limit their caffeine use.

Caffeine and the Prevention and Treatment of Stroke

A stroke is the sudden loss of consciousness, sensation, and ability to move that is caused by the obstruction (or sometimes the rupture) of an artery that normally brings blood to the brain. It can cause significant brain damage or death as brain cells, cut off from the blood supply, starve and die from lack of oxygen. Stroke can cause permanent neurological damage; complications and death can occur if not promptly diagnosed and treated. It is predicted that stroke will soon become the leading cause of death worldwide.

Regular consumption of caffeine can reduce the brain damage sustained from stroke. Caffeine protects the brain against the damage caused when a blood clot blocks blood flow. Studies have shown that clot-dissolving time is reduced by drinking coffee, but remains unaffected by drinking decaffeinated coffee. Researchers believe caffeine is the reason for the difference. Using caffeine regularly thus reduces the damage done if one suffers from a stroke.

The combination of alcohol content and caffeine in a beverage known as Irish coffee can offer significant protection against brain damage. If a person has had a stroke and they consume the Irish coffee soon enough they will be partially protected.

Recent studies by experts in the study of strokes show caffeine has neuroprotective functions. In studies done on animals, the combination of alcohol and caffeine showed over and over again a reduction in the damage to brain cells caused by strokes. The study showed that the combination reduced the tissue destroyed by over eighty-five percent.

Caffeine and alcohol didn't have the same effect on their own but only when they were combined. The combination seems to adjust the neurotransmitter systems just right. Another professor suggested it may be the antioxidant effects that account for the positive effects. As caffeine affects the regulation of certain receptors it may limit ischemic damage.

These studies done on the brains of certain animals were enough to excite the scientific community and assure further study will be done on this issue. There are enough similarities between the brains of rats and the brains of people for these results to merit such study.

Consider that with the right combination of alcohol and coffee they found that there's almost complete protection from a stroke. The results were both effective and striking. Unfortunately this combination is unlikely to be met with open arms by the pharmaceutical companies because these methodologies cannot be patented and such treatments would interfere with the sale of their more expensive drugs.

Caffeine and Surgery

Symptoms of caffeine withdrawal include depression, headache, muscles aches, and runny nose. These conditions can create trouble when a person abruptly stops using caffeine before an upcoming operation.

When a patient who normally consumes a cup of coffee in the morning doesn't have it they experience a headache upon waking from surgery due to the caffeine withdrawal. It is easy to combat the headache by simply giving the person the coffee upon awakening so long as that doesn't go against medical advice. Even if a person isn't allowed to drink yet, caffeine can even be given intravenously. This technique is being used in hospitals around the world to help patients combat these sometimes severe headaches. There are some doctors who even allow patients who use caffeine daily to have caffeine prior to surgery to avoid the headaches.

You can also avoid the headache situation if you eliminate caffeine from your diet gradually over the course of a few days prior to your surgery date.

Gallstone Disease and Caffeine

In recent study, men drinking two cups of coffee cut the risk of developing gallbladder disease nearly in half. The risk declined even more for those who drank four or more cups a day. The study was aimed at looking at the occurrence of new symptomatic gallstone disease, which can be detected by ultrasound and X-ray. This was part of a ten-year study done on the dietary habits of approximately sixty thousand men between the ages of thirty-five and eighty.

Researchers believe that caffeine, the active agent in coffee, was responsible for the protective effect, as the same results didn't occur with decaffeinated coffee.

Caffeine is able to help patients increase the flow of bile, while decreasing fluid absorption in the gallbladder. This is part of the way caffeine works to limit the risk of developing gallstones.

Caffeine and Asthma

Many children suffer from asthma. The primary symptoms of asthma are difficulty in breathing, wheezing, coughing, and thick mucus production. Many people need hospitalization after suffering from an asthma attack. For many years caffeine has been used to combat the symptoms of asthma because of its ability to relax the bronchial tissue and thus improve airway functioning.

Theophylline, a close relative of caffeine, has double the brochodilating potency of caffeine and can be found in many asthma medications. People with asthma who consume an average of two cups of coffee daily have an almost thirty percent fewer attacks. Caffeine is also used in this same capacity for treating newborns with neonatal apnea. This condition occurs most often in premature infants.

Heart Attacks and Caffeine

Homeostasis refers to the process whereby bleeding is halted, notably the body's coagulation process, or clotting. The process by which the body breaks down clots is known as fibrinolysis which averts thrombosis, a pathological condition in which a blood clot forms within a blood vessel. These clots can result in a stroke or heart attack.

There doesn't appear to be any effect on the coagulation process from caffeine or coffee consumption. Caffeine has shown in studies to increase the efficiency of fibrinolysis and thus help protect the heart against heart attacks. Caffeine appears to reduce clot-dissolving time. The results appear only in caffeinated coffee and not in the decaffeinated coffee, which suggests that caffeine is the responsible agent. If the theory is correct then caffeine operates in effectively the same way as many pharmaceutical products that are designed to reduce the risks of heart attacks and strokes.

Coffee and Smoking

Cigarettes increase the rate of caffeine metabolism, which may be one reason that smokers drink more coffee than non-smokers. Smokers must consume more caffeine to achieve the same effects as non-smokers. Therefore cigarette smokers who are eliminating tobacco should take into consideration the fact that caffeine will have a stronger effect on them once they are tobacco free. Caffeine will also last much longer once the tobacco has been eliminated. If someone who smokes was used to drinking one cup of coffee in the morning to get going he or she would probably need only half a cup once tobacco-free to get the same effect.

Another study found that if someone smokes a cigarette and consumes coffee at the same time, they will be partially protected against the development of chronic bronchitis and pulmonary edema. It appears that regular intake of coffee might be beneficial to smokers in delaying the development of lung disease. There needs to be more research done before anything definitive can be said, but the outlook is promising as to caffeine's ability to treat and even prevent pulmonary complications of smoking.

There has been recent research that suggests caffeine can help with lung disease caused by cigarette smoking. We know already that smokers can metabolize caffeine more rapidly than non-smokers. When a person smokes and drinks coffee the caffeine thus serves as a form of protection from some of the hazards of lung damage.

In treating premature infants suffering from apnea, the use of caffeine and caffeine-related substances has been affective. There are other drugs that have been used to treat this condition in infants, but physicians are using caffeine, theobromine, and theophylline more often now because they can manage the doses better, and it has a longer half-life than some of the other drugs previously used. They are actually exposed to less caffeine with the use of methylxanthine than some of the other drugs

Caffeine and Cancer

No disease inspires more fear in people than cancer. People are understandably afraid of anything that they hear may cause cancer. Caffeine has sometimes been called a carcinogen; and although there have been many studies that dismiss early reports that caffeine causes cancer the fear remains for some people.

Many of the studies conducted used coffee and not caffeine itself and because coffee contains so many active chemicals the studies need to be reevaluated. One study done on over thirty-five thousand people found no association between caffeine consumption and overall risk of cancer.

Caffeine can actually protect the body against certain types of cancer. Caffeine offers protection against certain tumor growths. Caffeine may well lessen the risk of developing some cancers. One study shows that maintaining a level of caffeine can have a deleterious effect on the development of breast cancer. Two separate studies showed that drinking three or four cups of coffee daily significantly reduced the incidence of breast cancer.

Coffee consumption has also been linked to combating colon cancer. The study showed a reduction of over twenty five percent in the occurrence of colorectal cancer amongst those drinking several cups of coffee daily compared with people not drinking any coffee. These studies were done on people from at least ten different countries. The overall conclusion was that caffeine inhibits cancer causing agents and protects against colon cancer. The study also showed a decrease in tumors.

Evidence suggests that perhaps it is the liver enzymes that metabolize caffeine, triggering carcinogenesis which essentially blocks the cancerous activity. Other foods with high levels of antioxidants also seem to combat cancer, which leads scientists to believe it is also the antioxidant power of caffeine that contributes to its cancer fighting ability.

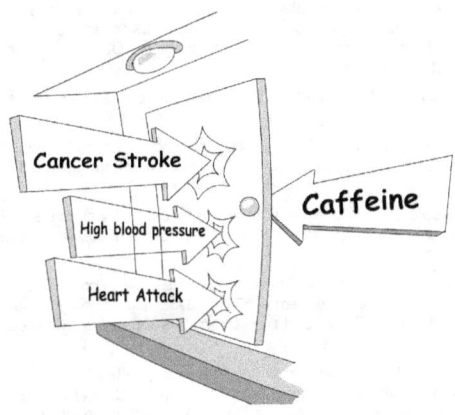

The possible relationship between coffee and cancer has been looked at in depth over the past few decades. We will look further at these studies and see if there is any light that can be shed on the relationship between caffeine and cancer.

Fibrocystic breast disease is a painful but otherwise harmless disease that causes many women to at first suspect breast cancer. Researchers have suspected a causal link between caffeine and this condition for many years. One study found no correlation between caffeine consumption and an increase in fibrocystic breast disease, while another showed that there was an increase of over 100 percent in women who consumed more than two cups of coffee daily. One researcher claimed that abstaining from caffeine could provide relief for two-thirds of women with fibrocystic breast disease.

Many other studies have concluded that there is not any link between caffeine use, and the incidence of cancers of the esophagus, stomach, liver, breast, ovaries or kidney.

Kids and Caffeine

One study showed that more than three quarters of infants tested positive for caffeine exposure at birth. Small children and adolescents consume less caffeine than adults but their exposure may be higher due to the concentration of caffeine in the body relativity to weight.

Another study showed that most children's average caffeine exposure compares to less than one cup of coffee daily. Like other studies we have discussed though there are many variables that need to be considered.

One study done a few decades back took into consideration many of these variables. This study found that almost twenty percent of infants less than two years old consumed some caffeine in any given two-week interval. In young infants they found that they were consuming as much caffeine as found in a cup of coffee containing seventy five milligrams per day. Infants are exposed to a much higher dose due to the immaturity of the infant's organs and their considerably smaller weight.

One recent study done on preschool age children found a correlation between high caffeine use and reports by parents of uncontrollable energy or hyperactivity, impulsiveness, headaches, restlessness, and other behavioral problems. All the symptoms are associated with attention deficit disorder (ADD), thus suggesting that many diagnoses of ADD may actually be misdiagnoses based on problems actually arising from caffeine use.

Another study concluded that caffeine may improve children's attention to detail and their manual dexterity and anxiety.

Caffeine is found in carbonated soft drinks, iced tea, and hot chocolate, which are popular drinks in young people. There is a huge void when it comes to information on the effect of caffeine on the young.

In most young people the predominate source of their caffeine was tea, soft drinks, and coffee. Chocolate foods and other beverages provided smaller amounts of caffeine but were a major source of dietary theobromine.

As more is known about the effects of caffeine, there is growing concern on how it affects children. There is also wide spread concern with any advertising campaigns that involve children and the use of caffeinated soft drinks. Certain research has shown children respond to the caffeine in soft drinks like an addictive drug.

Some studies showed that children experience withdrawal when they stop drinking soda and that they can be extremely sensitive to caffeine levels in soft drinks. Parents need to be aware that caffeine use can be habit forming and they need to pay attention to the way in which their child responds to caffeine.

Encouraging children to use pills of any kind is frowned upon by certain groups. One group that warns against the use of pills with caffeine in them is the "The Action for

Children's Television" (ACT). They have been successful at banning such ads. Now, makers of caffeine-based alertness aids are careful to target only an adult audience.

Caffeine: the Counterfeit Drug

Caffeine is often a component in amphetamine-based hallucinogens including; LSD, cocaine, and heroin; it is added to increase the psychoactive effects. The combination of caffeine and certain drugs is similar to a popular and extremely dangerous combination of heroin and cocaine called a "speedball."

During the 20th century there were cases of people distributing caffeine capsules that resembled "black beauties," also know as bathtub amphetamines. It was legal to purchase the caffeine pills however selling them was illegal. Customs officers have made drug busts and found large quantities of caffeine along with heroin and other illegal drugs and equipment to mix the two.

Rave parties are events where young people go to dance and often take many different drugs. They use a combination of potent psychedelics and stimulant drugs to help them stay awake in order to dance and party all night. The most commonly used drug at raves is ecstasy, a combination of several psychoactive drugs, LSD, and caffeine sometimes even heroin.

Reports of caffeine causing serious symptoms - including difficulty breathing and hallucinations from partygoers who end up in the hospital - have been circulating in the press. Tests showed that in some patients the key active ingredients were caffeine and an extract of the African kava root responsible for the hypnotic effect.

This case is more than likely a rare occurrence when it comes to the harm that young people incur at raves and with the use of ecstasy. I would suspect that caffeine is probably the least harmful thing they are ingesting. However it is important to be aware that the high levels of caffeine in some of these combinations can be dangerous.

More on Theophylline and Theobromine

Cacao contains eight times more theobromine than it does caffeine and has a smaller amount of caffeine than coffee by weight.

Theophylline is used more often for medical purposes than caffeine. Theophylline is not easily available, and where it does occur it is in minute quantities that have little effect. In order to have an effective dose it must be administered. It is used in inhalers for bronchodilation. Recently, over-the-counter drugs containing theopylline were declared unsafe and not effective by the Food and Drug Administration. Reports of serious side effects and even death have been linked to theophylline.

The combination of theophylline and ephedrine, which occurs in bronchodilator products and many cold medicines are often used for other purposes. There have been reports of teenagers using cold medicines to get high by drinking the entire bottle at once.

There have been attempts by the Food and Drug Administration to pull these products from the shelves because they are often used as weight control and muscle building aids without any proof of their true effect.

The three chemicals in coffee are all related but have very different profiles of action. The following is a brief summary of those three in order of significance.

Chemical:Caffeine
Sources:Coffee, tea, cola nuts, mate, guarana.
Effects: Stimulant of central nervous system, cardiac muscle, and respiratory system, diuretic.

Chemical:Theophylline
Sources: Tea
Effects: Cardiac stimulant, smooth muscle relaxant, diuretic, vasodilator.

Chemical:Theobromine
Sources: Cacao, also present in traces in cola nuts and tea.
Effects: Diuretic, smooth muscle relaxant, cardiac stimulant, vasodilator.

Caffeine and Birth Defects

The most recent recommendation of the medical and scientific community is that in order to avoid risk to the unborn fetus women shouldn't consume caffeine during pregnancy. There is conflicting evidence on this subject and many women use caffeine during pregnancy. This is shown in the fact that most babies are born with detectable levels of caffeine in their system. Fetal exposure to caffeine is possibly the cause of thousands of babies born with birth defects each year. It is very urgent that more investigation takes place on this subject to determine whether caffeine is responsible for these birth defects or if there is another responsible agent.

The livers of the fetus and newborn cannot metabolize caffeine. Due to this inability they cannot transform caffeine into its metabolites. This means the drug lingers in their systems much longer than it would in older children and adults. One study found that infants took almost fifteen times as long to eliminate the caffeine from their bodies than adults did, over ninety hours for some.

During the first months of life the capacity to metabolize caffeine increases dramatically. By around the ninth month of life it becomes almost equal to the adult level and does so by the end of the first year.

The fetus is at most risk for gross morphological abnormalities during the first three months of pregnancy, so the problem that occurs in the last three months shouldn't pose a great risk. The mother is less able to metabolize caffeine in the last trimester, but the fetus has passed the time when most abnormalities occur. Many recent reports exclude maternal caffeine use as a cause of gross morphological abnormalities in human infants.

Congenital abnormalities and defects are often associated with maternal exposure to drugs or chemicals. The fetus is much more vulnerable than either a child or an adult to the effects of drugs and chemicals. There are different risks at different stages of fetal development. The greatest risk for obvious deformations of the skeleton, face, or major organs occurs during the first three months of pregnancy. These are some of the reasons caffeine has been singled out for concern.

There is the possibility that caffeine interferes with the functioning or replication of genetic material. This possibility has given way to many studies on the subject. Caffeine would pose severe danger if in fact it does interfere with DNA. The danger would be most profound during the first weeks after conception because during this phase any damage done to the DNA could result in serious birth defects.

There hasn't been any evidence to demonstrate caffeine use causes adverse outcomes of pregnancy. However birth defects have consistently been found in laboratory animals that are exposed to "toxic" doses of caffeine. There is no proven relationship between maternal caffeine consumption and congenital skeletal malformations or malformations of organs found in human beings.

One study of more than fifty thousand pregnant women reported a small but significant dose-dependent increase in miscarriages. They suspect the increase is due to caffeine entering the egg just before the opportunity for implantation and causing the fertilized egg to get lost or develop abnormally.

In the later part of the 20th century doctors warned about dangers to fetal development if mothers were exposed to caffeine just prior to conception. The sperm cells were covered in a caffeine solution of fluctuating concentration. It is unknown exactly how this covering affects the egg.

Animal studies have also shown a link between behavioral abnormalities in the fetus and maternal use of caffeine. It is suspected that these same issues could occur in humans. However the studies done on humans have had conflicting results. One study showed no relationship between caffeine exposure on children and neurodevelopment, and another showed children had a greater arousal and irritability rate when exposed to caffeine.

Another prominent pediatrician investigated the effect coffee has on unborn babies. He found that within twenty minutes of the mother consuming coffee the fetus has more fetal movement. Another study showed caffeine intensified the contraction of the heart, and another showed that even low doses of caffeine can decrease placental blood flow.

It is common knowledge that anything ingested by the mother can cause an immediate reaction in the fetus. One example of this is in women who smoke. The study found a link between cigarette smoking and impaired or delayed response to stimuli in the fetus.

Caffeine and birth weight

Researchers have found a definite correlation between overweight mothers and overweight babies. Extra heavy babies cause delivery problems and are prone to childhood health problems. One factor linked to heavy babies was slow metabolism due to environmental and genetic factors. Caffeine will boost the metabolic rate of the child, minimize the size of fat cells, and program the body to burn fat. Four to six small (100 mg. of caffeine) cups per day are recommended. However, this is still controversial. More research needs to be done to weigh benefits and risks.

Babies Addicted to Caffeine?

Studies have been done to find out if the unborn fetus can become addicted to caffeine through exposure by the mother. One study showed that if the amount of caffeine consumed by the mother is high enough the baby will suffer withdrawal symptoms after birth. Children demonstrated unusual levels of irritability, jitteriness, and vomiting when mothers were heavy caffeine users. There is some evidence that suggests that caffeine withdrawal may cause neonatal apnea and sudden infant death syndrome (SIDS), as well as childhood diabetes.

If a mother uses caffeine while breast feeding the caffeine from her breast milk enters the infant's system. Because this is a time when the child metabolizes caffeine imperfectly, or not at all, the effect on the infant is multiplied many times. This means that the neurodevelopment can still be affected.

Even though there seems to be a legitimate reason to suspect danger to the infant, The American Academy of Pediatrics Committee on Drugs reported that moderate caffeine consumption has no effect on breast feeding. They suggest that both pregnant and nursing mothers use moderation when it comes to caffeine.

Caffeine's Effect on Fertility

Coffee has had a reputation for reducing fertility in men and women. It was before caffeine was ever isolated in coffee that these reports began. It was also suspected that coffee use reduces the libido in men and women. This was one reason that people used to argue against the use of coffee and coffeehouses during the 1600s. However, despite all the rumors, several studies have failed to find a connection between caffeine consumption and the risk of either delayed conception or infertility in women.

One study found that the amount of caffeine seemed to have no impact on the length of time it took women to conceive. It showed that on average it took around five months for women to conceive regardless of the amount of coffee they drank. They concluded that caffeine consumption was not a risk factor for primary infertility.

Yet other studies claim to show a link between caffeine consumption and delayed conception. It would stand to reason that women who are trying to conceive may want to limit the amount of caffeine they are consuming until a more clear answer is known.

The level of caffeine in seminal fluid correlates to the amount found in the blood. Caffeine seems to have some profound effects on the behavior of the sperm. When semen is exposed to high levels of caffeine immediately prior to artificial insemination, the increased motility is sufficient to double a woman's chances of getting pregnant.

However there is still question about the effects on the sperm that could later increase the occurrence of miscarriage. The studies seem to show that the effects of caffeine on sperm cells increase with the dose and then level off. Once they reach the leveling off point, increased doses have less impact, and the higher doses of caffeine can have the exact opposite effect. The studies seem to agree that if men drink one to two cups of coffee a day their sperm tends to have more density and mobility, but drinking more than two cups decreases sperm mobility and density. This is another area of study where the jury is still out.

Caffeine as a Laxative

Foods that are low in fiber can cause infrequent bowel movements, and because regular bowel movements remove toxic waste and speed weight loss this can be detrimental to one's health. In order to protect itself against harmful substances the body causes mucus to be formed in the colon long before the harmful food can reach it. The mucus lines the colon so that once the harmful substance reaches the colon it is prepared for elimination and the poison won't be absorbed. Then later it breaks down the substance and it exits the colon without causing any harm.

Over time, harmful foods are ingested that affects the colon's ability to function properly. The mucus lining in the bowel thickens. Layer piles upon layer and eventually there can be little room for waste to pass through.

Even in very young children rotting food and decaying fecal matter can be found. If a person has an unhealthy diet or suffers from constipation it can make matters even worse when it comes to colon function. The poor functioning colon results in a number

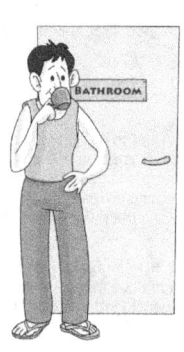 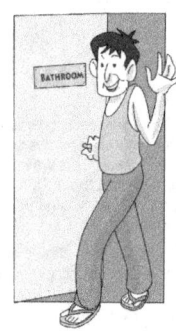

of different health problems. Many doctors suggest that it is okay to go a day or two with no bowel movement but this is not normal. A healthy person with a properly functioning digestive and elimination system should have 3 bowel movements a day. You may find it hard to believe that a normal bowel movement should be two inches across and two feet long.

A clean colon is very important. Toxins accumulate in the colon and they need to be eliminated from the body via the liver and kidneys. It is not recommended to use harsh chemical laxatives to cleanse the system. One of the best and most natural enemas is a coffee enema which you should use at least once a week. Another good thing to try is drinking aloe vera juice. There are many new products that contain wheat grass which help in detoxifying the liver. Using a combination of the wheat grass one week and a coffee enema the next week will greatly reduce the toxins in your liver.

Caffeine: the Colon Cleanser

According to one early writing, the enema is one of the longest used medical procedures in history. Enemas are injected into the rectum for the purpose of clearing out the bowel. In some countries enemas are used routinely on women and children.

One of the earliest known medical texts makes reference to using an enema calling it the "guardian of the anus." There were doctors were specialists in administering enemas to royals. The Egyptians in particular were known for their cleanliness. They believed that diseases were caused by bacteria from food waste in the body and shared this belief with others who came to their country.

Many countries knew about enemas in ancient times. It is reported that the Native Americans were responsible for the invention of an enema delivery system using parts of animal bladder and a hollow leg bone. Other countries used latex, creating the first rubber enema bags and tubes. Enemas are found throughout literature, even referenced in Shakespeare. The French were known to use enemas daily, and said it helped clear the skin as well.

Today, enemas are rarely used. Doctors still use them before and after surgeries and childbirth. Coffee has long been used for its medicinal qualities. It is unclear when it was first used for an enema, but it seems to have been in the early part of the 20th century. Scientists found that caffeine could be used to open the bile ducts. Caffeine could also be used to stimulate the production of bile in the liver. This held true with tests done on animals.

Doctors began experimenting with caffeine, using it as a detoxification regimen on patients with tuberculosis and cancer. Some remarkable effects were shown. Patients were able to rid themselves of pain-killers. Many patients reported a calming effect from the use of coffee enemas. The enemas can relieve constipation, but are used for the stimulation of the liver.

The coffee enema has been met with skepticism, but there has been some research that gives support to the theory that caffeine can stimulate the liver and thus discharge bile. A study showed caffeine promoted the activity of a key enzyme system which detoxifies a vast array of toxins from the bloodstream and thus could be used for carcinogen detoxification.

One study on animals showed that when coffee beans were included in the diet, the coffee enema showed a huge increase in the body's ability to rid itself of harmful carcinogens and other toxins.

The study found that cancer could not exist in normal metabolism, and in order to get a tumor to form it had to damage the thyroid. The detoxification systems are probably enhanced by the coffee enema, causing the excretion of toxic cancer breakdown products by the liver and dialysis.

Theophylline and theobromine found in coffee also dilate blood vessels and counter inflammation of the gut, which enhances the removal of toxic free radicals from the serum. The enemas perform a type of dialysis of blood across the gut wall.

There remains skepticism about coffee enemas, and many doctors hold the belief that not enough evidence supports the claim that coffee enemas detoxifies the blood or liver.

Caffeine and Longer Living

One study done at a highly regarded university in California showed that drinking one or more cups of coffee was associated with a significant reduction in all-cause mortality. The study also found that the same results were not true with an intake of calcium and other vitamins.

Caffeine, Blood Sugar, and Diabetes

Caffeine stabilizes blood sugar levels and triggers the release of chemicals that turn off the appetite center and halts food cravings. This stops binge eating in most people. Drinking coffee along with eating sweets spares the body the extreme swings n blood sugar when eating sweets alone.

A recent study has shown that the risk of diabetes was lowered by over thirty percent in those people who drank three or more cups of coffee a day. There seemed to be no benefits in people who drank any less than that per day.

Balzac on Caffeine

One great and prolific story-teller in history was unquestionably a caffeine addict. Balzac credited the effects of caffeine to coffee because he was unfamiliar with caffeine, which wasn't well known at the time. During his early years at school he smuggled in coffee beans and had a supply of his own. In his adult life he slept in the early evening and, rising at midnight, wrote his novels through the night, the next morning, and into the early afternoon. It was coffee which he consumed compulsively that made these all night writings possible.

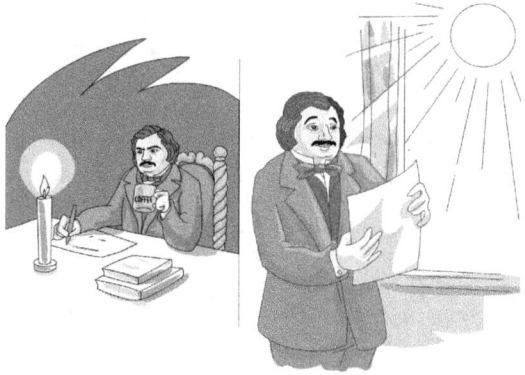

Like any true drug addict he believed he needed to use coffee in order to create his master pieces. He spoke of coffee's ability to keep him awake and also inspire his creative flow. But he also recognized the need to increase his "dose" to achieve the desired effects. He wrote "coffee is a great power in my life; I have observed its effects on an epic scale. . . . Many people claim coffee inspires them, but, as everybody knows, coffee only makes boring people even more boring."

He went on to talk about how coffee sets the blood in motion and acts as a muscle stimulant. He spoke of its ability to accelerate the digestive process and chase away sleep. He also noted that the length of time during which one can enjoy the benefits of coffee can be extended by changing the amount of coffee consumed. He found that if one grinds the coffee very thin with little water it would double the dose and one can continue working for several days.

He described another method using finely pulverized, dense coffee, cold and dry, consumed on an empty stomach. He suggested that using coffee in this method made one feel that everything became animated and ideas came quickly. He described a confused and highly alert state of mind which may be more rightly attributed to sleep deprivation than coffee, as at one point he thought he'd been poisoned and took to his bed.

Balzac suggested that under this condition a person should avoid going out in public as they may otherwise embarrass themselves. He speaks of coffee's effects much like that of other drugs:

being so heavily under the influence a person has to beware of where they go and who they talk to. He spoke of specific moments of socially unacceptable conduct induced by caffeine intoxication that became so embarrassing it kept him indoors whenever he drank coffee heavily thereafter.

He went on to speak of his increased tolerance and how he would resort to eating dry coffee powder. As with many other addicts, it would seem that this writer met his end early. The combination of abusing coffee and not getting enough sleep as well as working himself to the bone resulted in the writer having a weakened heart and ultimately he passed on.

CHAPTER TEN – WHEN A CUP ISN'T JUST A CUP

Coffee: Black as the devil, Hot as hell, Pure as an angel, Sweet as love.
~Charles Maurice de Talleyrand-Perigord

Many people assume that a "cup" of coffee is the same when reading research papers or other literature on coffee. This matter of what exactly constitutes a cup of coffee is another area where there are many variables to consider. Normally when referring to a cup of coffee we are talking about 100 mg. of caffeine.

One of the most obvious factors to consider in looking at the cup issue is the size of the cup being used. There are a variety of cups out there that people use every day for their morning coffee. Where one person's container may be a Styrofoam cup at the office; another may have a favorite coffee mug that is twice the size. Another problem is how much of the cup is being filled with coffee. It may be normal for one person to only fill their coffee cup half way while another fills it to brim. This can create a situation where one person is getting 2-4 ounces on average per cup and other is getting 10-12 ounces. The next factor to look at is how much caffeine is in the coffee being used. This is dependent on what types of beans are being used as well as how the coffee is being prepared.

The problem that arises is where one small cup of weaker coffee may contain less than 100 mg. of caffeine, while another larger cup with stronger caffeine content may contain over 300 mg. of caffeine. It is most commonly found that people get between 100-250 mg. of caffeine per cup. However the point we are making is that there is much room for error in these numbers.

The same problems faced in looking at a "cup" of coffee hold true when it comes to tea. There are few studies that have been done to look closely at the caffeine content in tea and coffee served in restaurants, cafes, and coffee shops. There is also a lack of research done on the caffeine content of coffee prepared at home.

There was a study done in the later part of the 1980s that looked at over sixty-five different locations where coffee was prepared. They found a large difference in comparison of caffeine content from location to location. They also showed even from day to day in the same location the caffeine content could change considerably. The range was anywhere from less than 20 mg to over 400 mg. per cup. Another interesting note was that most decaffeinated coffee served in retail outlets actually contained caffeine upon further examination.

There were several different brands of instant coffee that were studied and it was found that there was a considerable amount of variation in caffeine content as well. The same tests were done on tea and they showed very similar results.

Caffeine in Tea

In tea, the caffeine content is largely dependent on the age of the leaves and the manner in which they were cured. Ma-Cha tea, which is often used in the Japanese culture, has the highest caffeine content of all teas. It is made from tiny leaves of newly budding plant. Herb and mint teas on the other hand are made from plants that don't contain caffeine. The following three factors can affect how much caffeine is present in a cup of tea:

Length of fermentation
   A. Green tea, which is unfermented, has the least caffeine
   B. Oolong, which is partially fermented, has about 50 percent more
   C. Black tea, which is fully fermented, has three times as much.

The length of brewing time.
   A. Black tea infused for three minutes has 20 to 40 mg.
   B. black tea infused for four minutes has 40 to 100 mg.

The amount of caffeine in leaf powder.
   A. Caffeine found in tea bags is more readily dissolved in water and will on average have almost twice the caffeine as higher-quality full-leaf tea.

Caffeine in Decaf?

Trying to determine how much caffeine is in the coffee we order at restaurants or cafes it is virtually impossible. One study showed a 100% variation in caffeine content served in such places. It was a surprise to learn that similar discrepancies were noted in another study done on the decaffeinated coffees served at some of the most popular coffeehouses in the world. Looking at several different samples, they found an average of at least 10 mg. of caffeine in decaffeinated coffee. The leading coffee chain (Starbucks) had twice as much.

The following chart was developed from data found in several different studies that were conducted using cups that contained at least 8 ounces of liquid.

The large fluctuation in caffeine content explains why sometimes you get just the kick you need from only one cup of coffee and other times it takes several cups to get the same results. Take into consideration there is of course some room for error in the following chart, but it was created from the results of several different scientific studies.

Brand	Milligrams found in a 6 oz. serving
Starbucks decaffeinated	22-25
Dunkin' Donuts decaffeinated	10-12
Starbucks decaffeinated espresso	6-9
McDonald's decaffeinated	2-5
7 - Eleven decaffeinated	2-5
Tetley decaffeinated tea	2-5
Dalton's decaffeinated	2-5
Sanka	0-2

As we mentioned earlier, the amount of caffeine in the individual beans affects the caffeine content in a cup of coffee. Ironically the more expensive Arabica beans have less than half the caffeine content of cheaper Robusta beans. The Arabica beans have more lipids than the Robusta beans but they are otherwise similar when it comes to the minerals, proteins, and carbohydrates.

Mate and Caffeine Content

The age and time of harvest greatly affects the amount of caffeine in mate. Mate is a significant source of caffeine. It is difficult to determine the exact levels of caffeine in mate because there are over sixty varieties of plants that can be used to make the drink. The older leaves have slightly less caffeine that younger leaves. As the leaves age they gradually lose the amount of caffeine.

Guarana and Caffeine Content

Guarana is another source of caffeine often found in herbal elixirs and powders in health food stores. Most guarana capsules contain about 25 mg. of caffeine. As with coffee, there are different active alkaloids that affect the way people react to beverages containing guarana. It is similar to coffee and mate in the sense that it is also very difficult to determine the caffeine content.

Chocolate

There is very little caffeine found in chocolate and other products made from cacao. The typical Hershey bar for example on has about 12 mg. of caffeine and a cup of hot chocolate has about 5 mg. of caffeine.

Soft Drinks

The amount of caffeine in soft drinks varies widely from brand to brand. We will look at few different brands and the amount of caffeine in them in the following chart:

Brand	Caffeine content
Red Bull	80 mg.
Jolt	70 mg.
Mountain Dew	55 mg.
Mello Yellow	52 mg.
Coca Cola	46 mg.
Pepsi	37 mg.
7-Up	0 mg.

Caffeine in Over-the-Counter Drugs

There are over one thousand different over-the-counter medications that use caffeine. Caffeine can be found in the following four categories: analgesics, cold remedies, appetite suppressants, and diuretics. Caffeine is also the only active ingredient in many pills used for alertness aids. Two of the most popular contain anywhere from 100-200 mg. per pill.

Theobromine and Tehophylline in Caffeinated Beverages

Theobromine and theophylline are found in all of the caffeine sources mentioned above. Because each has a different profile the effects of each can be different. Theobromine is a more potent diuretic than either caffeine or theophylline. Theophylline is often used as a bronchodilator. Cacao, being a major source of theobromine, also contains small amounts of caffeine. The total methylxanthine in cacao will vary from plant to plant.

Mate leaves also have a small amount of these methylxanthines, which are almost undetectable. In addition to caffeine, theobromine, and theophylline, tiny amounts of other purine alkaloids can be found in coffee.

A Final Word of Advice

As we can see here the amount of caffeine in the most popular caffeinated beverages can vary greatly from cup to cup. Unless you are already taking a caffeine pill in which you know the exact caffeine content, it is best to experiment with other caffeinated beverages until you find the right dose. In order to avoid any problems you may want to start with a smaller dose and take note to how it affects your overall energy level and appetite.

CHAPTER ELEVEN – DISPELLING THE MYTHS ABOUT CAFFEINE

I have measured out my life with coffee spoons. ~T.S. Eliot

There are many myths about caffeine, some of which we have touched on in previous chapters. We will take a closer look here at that folklore.

1) Caffeine increases anxiety.
2). Caffeine raises blood pressure.
3). Caffeine is bad for your heart.
4).Caffeine causes dehydration.

Does Caffeine Cause or Increase Anxiety?

In some studies caffeine has been shown to provoke panic attacks in people with panic disorder. In addition, these studies have concluded that caffeine may increase anxiety and cause insomnia. The effects of caffeine seem to vary widely from individual to individual; anxiety disorder specialists often recommend that people with panic disorder eliminate all caffeine consumption. Other research, however, shows that this belief is a misconception. The truth is, most people who use caffeine actually experience lower levels of anxiety than people who do not. Very large doses of caffeine can slightly increase anxiety levels in some people. Small to moderate doses of caffeine usually have a relaxing or tranquilizing effect.

Confusing Results with Blood Pressure

In people who don't consume caffeine on regular basis, caffeine can cause a temporary elevation in blood pressure. Some researchers suggest the elevation is caused by caffeine narrowing the blood vessels and blocking the effects of adenosine. Caffeine may also stimulate the adrenal gland to release more adrenaline, which would also cause your blood pressure to increase.

Some research has found that people who regularly drink caffeine have a higher average blood pressure than those who drink none. As they build a tolerance to it, however, caffeine doesn't appear to have a long-term effect on their blood pressure.

Yet another study done over a ten year period on more than 150,000 females found that drinking caffeinated cola may be associated with an increased risk of high blood pressure. Yet, the same causal relationship was not found with caffeinated coffee. In fact, the study suggested that women who drink caffeinated coffee may actually have a reduced risk of high blood pressure.

A more recent study claims that women who drink six cups of caffeinated coffee a day have lower risks of high blood pressure. Some doctors recommend limiting caffeine to 200 milligrams a day. They also recommend avoiding caffeine right before activities that naturally increase your blood pressure.

Can Caffeine Cause Hypertension?

Several studies have examined tens of thousands of individuals considered at high risk for developing hypertension and other heart conditions. Time and time again they have shown no link between caffeine intake and the incidence of high blood pressure or heart disease of any sort.

Studies also show that while there might be a slight rise of blood pressure at first, this effect dissipates quickly as a person develops a tolerance to caffeine.

The consumption of hot beverages, whether they contain caffeine or not, seems to increase both diastolic and systolic blood pressure. They also increase the heart rate, which produces a greater increase than that produced by caffeine ingestion alone. This may be one reason may for some reports attributing transient blood pressure effects to caffeine.

The Dehydration Myth

Research has proven that caffeine is not responsible for causing dehydration. Caffeine seems to have no diuretic effect at all on people, whether they are at rest or are vigorously exercising. This is another myth which probably got started because drinking hot fluids has a diuretic effect. The caffeine in coffee does not contribute to this effect but the heat of the beverage does.

Dehydration often occurs when traveling on a plane, but the cause has nothing to do with whether a person uses caffeine or not. It is caused by cabin air that is extremely dry in most planes.

The truth is, many people use caffeine to fight off sleepiness and fatigue while traveling: by road or by air. The use of caffeine can no doubt help travelers cope with jet lag. An even better way to avoid these problems is using a well-thought-out program that helps maximize all the benefits that caffeine can offer if used properly. These programs will be discussed in more detail in later chapters.

Bad Advice About a Good Drug

The notion that anything that makes you feel good must be bad in some way is ingrained in most peoples' consciousness. Caffeine is a mood-altering drug that supports a physical dependence; as such it is often associated with other much harder and dangerous drugs. People often think if it's a drug than it must be immoral and there are serious physical or mental side effects.

We've looked at reports since the nineteenth century when caffeine was thought to cause a depletion of our energies and a great plummet after it was metabolized.

The body gets its energy by burning food, and caffeine increases our metabolism and the rate at which we burn fat. If caffeine isn't interfering with your sleep, then there is no downside to using it. Some scholars suggest caffeine upsets our balance; however caffeine is actually a great restorer of the balance of our neurotransmitter systems.

There can be a risk of caffeine dependency. It is simple though to avoid this pitfall by following the guidelines that will be laid out for you in our program.

Caffeine is safe, reliable, non-toxic, easily monitored, and the body does not build up a great tolerance to it. One early writer on coffee was quoted as saying, "Give a man enough coffee and he's capable of anything."

When used properly caffeine can truly help us achieve our physical, metal and weight goals. In previous chapters gave you the basic information you need to understand the dynamics of caffeine's effects. It is important to pay attention to any side effects and physical dependence issues as results vary from person to person. We use the old saying that "less is more" because a small to moderate doses of caffeine can often do more good than a larger one.

Some of the advantages we gain can help us succeed at work and even save our lives on the highway. The invention of the light bulb brought about late nights at the office. This advance in technology is linked with a disruption of the 24-hour daily rhythm. Most people do not even realize that their body actually operates on a twenty-five, rather than a twenty-four hour schedule. Caffeine can help use remain on a 25-hour cycle.

More Benefits

Caffeine can actually be used to improve sleep. Studies have proven its ability to elevate intelligence and memory. Artists have known for centuries that caffeine can enhance creativity. It is also a great social lubricant that is known for improving our interactions.

In the following chapters we will look further into caffeine's ability to enhance physical performance and endurance. The results are equally astonishing in the way caffeine aids in weight loss and dieting. We will also provide evidence that caffeine can help prevent aging, and even counteract certain diseases. There is no question that caffeine has become the favorite and most important recreational drug of the twenty-first century.

CHAPTER TWELVE - CAFFEINE AND WEIGHT LOSS

Nancy Astor: "If I were your wife, I would put poison in your coffee."
Sir Winston Churchill: "And if I were your husband, I would drink it."

Separating Fact From Fiction

The modern day Holy Grail is the "fat pill." There are hundreds of genetics companies, scientists, and universities searching for a safe, pharmacologically active compound that can be used to contain appetite, reduce hunger, and minimize fat retention. On the market today are thousands of different diet aids, but none that really works well for long term weight loss. Once the perfect "fat pill" is discovered the persons responsible will certainly be rewarded as the gods of Greek mythology were.

There are many such aids that do work at suppressing appetite and increasing the metabolism. The problem with these "aids" is that most of them are illegal and very unsafe. There has been little success in finding a pill that works at keeping weight off while being safe in the long run.

These aids help burn fat at a faster rate, but they lose effect as usage continues. Many amphetamine derivatives have been used legally in prescription drugs for decades. Today they are being prescribed less and less for weight loss or obesity treatment. There has been a revolution of sorts in the world of natural medicine when it comes to diet aids. All types of "natural" products boast the ability to burn fat and speed up one's metabolism. Most people are smart to be skeptical about the ability of such drugs to really do all the things in which advertisements claim they can.

There is one amazing drug however that can truly and safely accomplish all the things that scientists seem to be looking for in the perfect diet pill. That amazing drug is caffeine.

A highly-respected and well-known researcher wrote about many of the remarkable effects of caffeine. He stated that in addition to the many other helpful affects on the body, caffeine affects the fat tissue by stimulating lipolysis. He noted caffeine's ability to increase the catabolism, or burning of fat. He also spoke of caffeine's role in blocking the effect of adenosine and adenosine analogs, which enables the body to burn fat faster and allow a person to lose weight.

There is a vast amount of evidence to support these findings. In studies conducted on people while they are exercising, the effects of caffeine were profound. Time and time again researchers found that when people used a heavy dose of caffeine prior to exercising they lost significantly more weight than those who did not ingest caffeine. The level of fatty acids released from the adipose tissue is greatly increased by caffeine use.

Studies show that it takes approximately four hours for caffeine to enhance fat oxidation. Runners and other athletes have used caffeine for many years to enhance fatty acid metabolism. Several studies conducted on this subject suggest that the benefits are most profound during longer duration exercise that is less intense. In this type of exercise the body's lipids have a more important role in energy production. The effects are generally only really noticed by people who are "weekend warriors."

There are other ways in which caffeine contributes to weight loss. In both overweight and average weight people, caffeine has been shown to increase the base and resting metabolic rate by over 10 percent. The effect appears to last for a few hours after caffeine is ingested.

The Pounds Add Up

There are hundreds of books written about weight loss, attempting to find the answer for how people can lose weight and why they gain it in the first place. There is a simple answer to these complex questions. The amount of calories you burn in comparison to the amount of calories you take in determines whether you gain or lose weight.

It is estimated that a person will gain half a pound for every 1750 calories that they take in but fail to burn off. Likewise, if you burn 1750 calories without adding calories o your diet, you will lose one half of a pound. If you repeatedly take in approximately 100 more calories per day than you burn than you will gain approximately ten extra pounds per year. Calories can be burned by exercising and doing work but they are also burned by simple activities like breathing.

Your metabolism is the major factor in how slow or fast you burn calories. The slower your metabolism the fewer you calories you burn in a given time period. There are some who seem to get away with murder when it comes to the amount of food they eat without gaining any weight. This would be a person with a fast metabolism.

The major ways calories are burned consists of the three following:

A. The energy you use just by breathing, circulating blood, and staying warm accounts for 40-80 percent of your calories you burn.
B. Digestion accounts for between 5-15 percent of your calories. This happens as a result of the way the body processes the food it ingests.
C. Physical activity accounts for 10-35 percent. This can be any physical activity, from simply walking out to get the mail to running a marathon.

How Caffeine Influences the Metabolic Rate

Caffeine aids in weight loss because it causes a person to burn more calories than they would otherwise. A slight increase or decrease in metabolism can have enough impact on a person to determine whether they lose or gain weight; whether they are fat or thin. Caffeine appears to affect the neuro-transmitter systems and increases the metabolic rate by releasing catecholamines.

One study showed that if a person consumed about two cups of coffee, their metabolism was increased by nearly 20 percent and last over 120 minutes. Over time, these small changes add up to pounds, and the pounds add up. Even if a person is burning an extra 200 calories a day, that can turn into a loss of twenty pounds over a period of a year.

Now, keep in mind two factors. 1) These figures are based on drinking three cups of coffee a day. On our program, we recommend six cups of coffee over the course of a day. 2) Coffee triggers the release of CCK which signals the hypothalamus, suppressing the appetite.

Just How Good is Caffeine at Calorie Burning?

The following is a way to find out how many calories you can burn using caffeine. First you must find out your basal metabolic rate. You can use the following equation to get an estimate:

1. Multiply your weight in pounds by 4.4
2. Multiply your height in inches by 4.7
3. Add 1 and 2.
4. Multiply your age in years by 4.7
5. Subtract 4 from 3
6. Add 655 plus 10 percent.
7. Take 10 percent of this amount. This will tell you about how many extra calories you can burn by increasing your metabolic rate just 10 percent with caffeine. Remember that the 10% rate is based on three cups of coffee a day. On the Caffeine Diet, you will be drinking 6 cups per day.

How to Maximize Caffeine's Benefits

One way, of course, is to increase the total amount of caffeine we are taking daily. The other way is to consume caffeine at the proper times. If, for example, a person was to take a caffeine pill prior to eating lunch, this would suppress appetite by up to 30%. The greater asset is caffeine's ability to suppress appetite. We will look much closer at this in the following pages.

When a person is tired, their metabolic rate slows. Caffeine counteracts this effect and boosts a person's metabolism so they are equal to that of a well rested person's. Caffeine also works to restore energy and improve one's mood.

The main question people want to know is, "Does caffeine really work as an effective aid in the battle of the bulge, and if so just how exactly does it help? The answer of course is "yes" and we will look at exactly how it does so.

Countless studies have been done on the relationship between caffeine and exercise. The focus is on how caffeine effects fax oxidation. There are many variables to integrate into any formula, including:

1. How much caffeine is consumed.
2. How long before the test is it consumed.
3. How long the exercise is continued.
4. The physical condition of the subject.
5. The tolerance of the subject to caffeine.
6. Which muscles are being used in the exercise.
7. Any relative psychogenic effects.

Caffeine Suppresses Appetite

We've discussed in earlier chapters how caffeine works like other stimulants as an anorectic, or appetite suppressant. Consuming caffeine prior to eating suppresses the feeling of hunger and also minimizes the amount of food it takes in order to feel full. It is the habit of many people to enjoy a cup of coffee after a meal, however adding a cup before can have far more positive benefits.

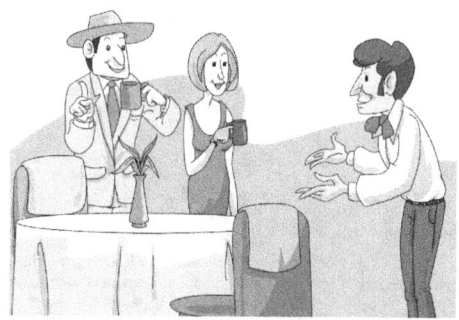

Due to the fact that people react to coffee in different ways, a person should experiment in order to find the right levels needed to gain the maximum benefit. It is better to start with a smaller amount like 50 milligrams (3 oz. of drip coffee). Remember that the caffeine found in tea has a different effect than that of coffee. There are other agents at work in coffee that promote benefits not found in tea.

Caffeine is more a way of life than a fact of life. It offers a wide array of benefits far superior to any other drug in the pharmacopoeia. In order to really use caffeine strategically it is important to understand the scientific studies that have revealed some of the many benefits of caffeine use.

Caffeine as a Diet Aid

We want to drive home the point that it is always important to experiment because individual responses can vary considerably.

There is evidence of caffeine's ability to work as a diet aid throughout history. Early accounts speak of the natural sources of caffeine to stave off hunger. Ancient warriors carried balls of fat mixed with crushed coffee beans to help fight off hunger during battle.

Caffeine as an appetite suppressant has stood the test of time. Both ancient and modern science, confirm that caffeine is an anorectic. There have been numerous studies done on animals that leave little room for doubt about this quality. One study showed that when rats were administered the equivalent of 300 mg. of caffeine their appetite was suppressed by 35% to 95%. There haven't been as many studies done on humans but all the animal studies so far agree on the matter.

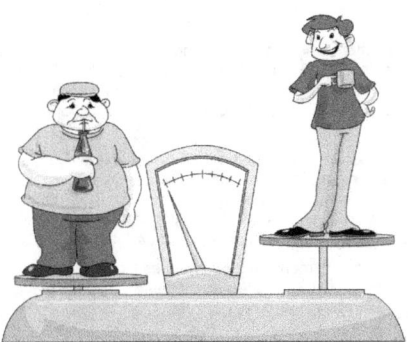

The large doses of caffeine had such dramatic affects on reducing hunger that it leads one to conclude small doses must have a similar, though less dramatic, affect. As we mentioned, simply reducing your food intake by ten percent will lead to dramatic weight loss over time.

Anorexia and Caffeine

The disease anorexia nervosa typically affects young women who are pathologically afraid of gaining weight. They become unwilling to eat even when they are dying of starvation; they believe no matter how thin they are that they aren't thin enough. Studies done on a group of anorexic patients found that they admitted to using caffeine to stave off hunger, and the result was they could get by with eating nearly nothing.

The patients admitted that they consumed many highly-caffeinated beverages in order to increase energy and suppress appetite. Some patients admitted to drinking nearly one gallon of caffeinated beverages a day.

This example, not withstand how recklessly caffeine was used, does demonstrate its effectiveness in fighting off hunger and working as a diet aid. Of course we would never suggest using it in the manner in which the anorexic patients used it.

Caffeine and Serotonin

The way in which caffeine regulates serotonin levels is thought to be one key to its appetite-suppressing power. When a person has low serotonin levels they may feel hungry and melancholy at the same time.

There are many drugs on the market today that work at increasing serotonin levels to combat depression and anxiety. The affect of consuming foods that have high carbohydrate levels is similar. The problem with that is you are gaining weight because carbohydrates contain so many calories (and also trigger an insulin reaction which further stimulates appetite). The solution is simple: caffeine achieves the same effect minus the high calorie intake.

The Snowball Effect

It is very common to eat more when you are feeling depressed. The snow ball effect of course is that often times the more depressed a person is the more they eat. The more they eat the more weight they are going to gain. Feeling depressed because of weight gain will lead most people to unfortunately eat more to get rid of the depressed feeling; this is a never ending cycle for millions of people every day.

There truly is a much easier way to break the cycle of depression. Caffeine is known for its ability to boost the mental and emotional spirits along with the extra energy it provides. It seems a logical solution to fighting off depression. These effects increase the likelihood a person will exercise, and exercise itself increases endorphins and provides a natural high. This combination can truly help a person avoid spiraling downward into depression.

Coffee stimulates the release of many potent hormones, some of which are natural appetite-suppressants like cholecystokinin (CCK). Coffee stimulates the release of this hormone and thus helps to create a feeling of fullness.

More simply put, caffeine makes a person feel full much quicker than they otherwise would. Caffeine also works to keep that feeling of fullness last. One experiment used the leaves of highly-caffeinated plants to create an elixir. Over a month and a half there was significant weight loss in the patients. Not only did they lose weight, but following the patients afterward showed that most were able to keep the weight off. Anyone who has struggled with dieting knows that keeping the weight off is the greater part of the battle.

Dexadrine

One prescription drug in the 1960s called Dexedrine contained dextroamphetamine. People were using Dexedrine to suppress appetite and increase energy, and it appeared to be the new wonder drug for a while. What we later learned was the drug was highly addictive and many people, young and old, became hooked on the drug.

Dextroamphetamine, like other illegal stimulants, produces dependency in people that cause them to increase the dosage to higher and higher levels. Patients were demanding from their doctors more and more of the medication even though they were told to only use it for a few weeks. Unfortunately many doctors gave in to patients and kept prescribing the drug. It took some time, but eventually the FDA recognized the dangers with Dexedrine being used for weight loss and they put a stop to things. .

Caffeine and losing the right fat

Caffeine not only helps you lose weight, but it helps you lose the right weight! Let's take a look at the different types of fat and how caffeine consumption affects those. The three types of fat are:

1) Structural Fat
2) Normal Fat Reserves
3) Abnormal Fat Reserves

Structural Fat: surrounds the organs and joints of the body. It protects them by providing cushion under the bones and also keeps the skin smooth and tight.

Normal Fat: Normal fat is the fuel of the body which is spread all over. This fat helps the body to deal with any insufficiencies when it comes to nutrition and calorie intake. These normal fat reserves are important to maintain overall good health. Typically when people diet or do exercise programs to lose weight it is the normal fat and structural fat which is lost. This type of weight loss accounts for many people suffering muscle and joint pain during the process because they are losing important normal fat reserves as well as muscle mass.

Abnormal Fat: Abnormal fat is located in specific areas more prone to fat storage. In females these area are the hips, thighs, and buttocks. In men the areas affected arenthe waist and upper chest. This type of fat is used for survival. It is only released in the most nutritional emergencies when the body is nearing starvation. These fat stores are also released during gestation for the survival of the unborn fetus. In people who are overweight most of the fat is stored in the areas mentioned, which creates the disfiguration we see in obese people. This also creates a situation where it is almost impossible for obese people to lose weight. However there is one substance that helps burn the abnormal fat, and that is caffeine.

Caffeine and Abnormal Fat

A problem many obese people face when trying to lose weight is that they are left feeling weak and extremely hungry. This is because they are losing the structural fat and normal fat. They are unable to lose the fat in the places they most want to such as the hips, thighs, buttocks, belly and upper arms. Often times, they even begin to look older and show more visible signs of aging like wrinkles as they lose the structural fat but retain the abnormal fat. This results in obese patients feel worse when they lose weight than they do if they gain or stay the same weight.

In fact, when obese people try to increase physical activity and reduce calories they end up actually gaining weight. This is because the metabolic rate is falling faster than the calories consumed are.

The Problem With Most Diets

When a person is lucky enough to lose weight when dieting they are really only losing water, muscle, and structural fat. These diets tend to increase your appetite, while at the same time lowering your metabolism. This situation eventually causes the body to store excess fat in the areas we discussed earlier.

Even in people who don't start out being what is considered obese, become that way after failing on successive diets. Here's why: if you go on a diet program for one year, cutting your caloric intake from 2400 to 1200 calories, you will then gain weight when you consume 1200 calories. This may be why nearly 95% of people doing any form of a conventional diet fail. It all has to do with how the metabolism is slowed and the problems that arise from that.

The Skinny on Caffeine and Metabolism

Highly refined food is served in about 95% of all fast food restaurants. A large percent is actually super highly refined. Trans-fats, which are anything hydrogenated or partially hydrogenated, or high fructose corn syrup, are found in almost every item served in those establishments. This is one of many reasons why an astonishing 80% of Americans are considered overweight and 50% are considered obese. You may have heard different figures, like 33% obese and 66% overweight. But those figures are based on new standards adopted in 2000 to make us seem less fat. If we go by 1950 standards, then we see the true picture.

These refined foods cause the hypothalamus to operate abnormally. Also, these types of trans fats are deposited in the problem areas mentioned above.

Another reason many people fail when following such programs is that naturally thin people and those who are obese have bodies that operate in considerably different ways. The overweight person has a very slow metabolism and thin people generally have a normal or faster metabolism. The result of this difference in metabolism creates a situation where both people eat the same amount of food but only the overweight person would gain weight.

When you have a slow metabolism your body cannot burn the food as fuel and thus it is converted into fat. In order for a person to rapidly lose weight they must have a normal or fast metabolism. Once this happens they can eat virtually whatever they want without gaining weight. The Caffeine Diet is the only method known that really resolves this problem.

Curing the Intense Hunger Pangs

Obese people feel a true, constant, and intense hunger that causes them to eat more than thin people. It is not because they lack will power or are weak people, but is due to how they react to food. The taste, texture, and smells trigger intense and consistent cravings. When overweight people eat a normal portion they do not feel satisfied or full. This feeling of being hungry lasts longer than it does in thin people and they wind up eating more . . . much more.

In thin people, the hunger mechanism shuts off much quicker and the feeling of hunger is low or even nonexistent for many hours after eating small quantities of food. In other diet plans there is no way of addressing the intense hunger in overweight people.

In order to have any success at all in losing weight this condition must be corrected. The Caffeine Diet does this. Overweight people tend to eat foods that create problems. When a person feels extremely hungry they usually have low blood sugar. So they reach for foods that will provide an immediate sugar replacement, regardless of whether or not they are healthy for them. Once on the Caffeine Diet, the intense hunger pangs and cravings will disappear and you will have the will power to choose foods that are good for you. On the Caffeine Diet you can eat virtually anything you want; you just won't eat as much. You will also no longer crave certain types of foods so intensely. This is the first step in being set free from the slavery created by uncontrollable cravings that many overweight people have lived with for so long.

Genetics and Obesity

Genetics determine basic body shape and structure. We know genetics determine what color eyes a person will have or if they will be short or tall. Genetics, however, play a relatively small role when it comes to obesity. It is true that some people are just naturally wider and thicker but that doesn't mean they are destined to be overweight.

Caffeine has been used successfully by tens of thousands of people for decades, even centuries if we accept old records. The Caffeine Diet can and will correct a low metabolism and insure success in reaching your weight goals.

Beyond an Under active Thyroid: What Else Causes Low Metabolism

Looking at symptoms and the causes for each symptom we will eventually get to the root of the problem. This is vital when dealing with any problem physical or mental. In business or personal life this is a way to truly resolve the problems that need to be addressed rather than just put a band-aid on them.

Having an under active thyroid is the number one cause of low metabolism. The other reason is a hypothalamus gland that functions improperly. We have already looked at the first cause, the thyroid. Now we will take a closer look at this second cause.

The following is a list of many variables that can affect the hypothalamus: having a clogged colon or liver, using artificial sweeteners, eating to many trans fats, too many food additives, growth hormones and antibiotics in food, lack of sun and sleep, nutritional deficiencies, eating pasteurized food, eating genetically modified food, lack of walking, non-prescription and prescription drugs, chlorine from the water you drink and bathe in, high fructose corn syrup, chemicals introduced into the body through the skin in the form of lotions and creams, carbonated drinks. These are just some of the causes so as you can see there are many reasons for improper functioning of the hypothalamus.

What Causes problems for the Hypothalamus?

1. Genetics. It is true that everyone is born with different metabolic rates. People are born with naturally high metabolisms and abnormally low metabolisms every day. But as we will learn, genetics are not carved in stone. There are steps we can take to ignite our metabolic rate.

2. A clogged liver. Nearly every overweight person when tested has been shown to have a clogged liver. This may occur from the over use of non-prescription and prescription drugs, the consumption of trans fats, including hydrogenated oils, artificial sweeteners, which are so common place in many foods today. One thing we know is that having a clogged liver will ensure that a person will have a low metabolism and store fat rather than burn it. We also know that caffeine causes the liver to flush more often, defending the body against this outcome.

3. Candida yeast. There is good and bad bacteria in your colon. Taking antibiotics destroys the good bacteria and allows bad bacteria like Candida yeast to over grow, which clogs the colon. Once the colon is clogged we know metabolism slows and bloating and gas build up. It also creates food cravings for bread, pasta, cheese, and sugar.

4. A clogged colon. We mentioned earlier that if a person is not having at least three bowel movements each day they have a clogged colon. There are many reasons the colon gets clogged: using non-prescription and prescription drugs, lack of water, fiber, and exercise. There can be many pounds of fecal matter in the colon. Until it is cleaned, digestion remains slow, and because nutrients are poorly absorbed, hunger will remain high.

5. Lack of enzymes. Food that comes from a jar or can have been pasteurized, which kills all the enzymes in the food. Microwaving food also kills the enzymes. Even most

fruits and vegetables today are devoid of enzymes because of the gassing used in the ripening process and the irradiation process. This lack of enzymes causes gas, bloating, constipation, and slow digestion.

6. Inefficient pancreas. People with a weight problem have a pancreas that is not operating properly and have insulin tolerance problems. Some factors are: drugs, artificial sweeteners, corn syrup. If this problem isn't corrected the body will store more fat.

8. Hormonal imbalances. Hormonal imbalances are caused by stress and chemical additives.

9. Artificial sweeteners. All man-made artificial sweeteners slow metabolism.

10. Lack of water. A lack of pure water hydrating the cells causes a lower metabolic rate. Most people are dehydrated and are unaware of it.

11. Carbonated drinks. Soft drinks cause weight gain due to the way the brain reacts to sweet tastes, sending false messages to the liver. When the sugar that was promised by the taste buds is nowhere to be found, the brain and liver panic and signal the body to secure sugar or simple carbs quickly.

12. Lack of sleep. Anything less than seven hours of sleep per night is considered a lack of sleep. The brain thinks you are staying awake longer because there is danger and thus goes into the fight or flight response. This reaction signals the hypothalamus that we need food. Also, the body, for reasons not yet known, processes sugar improperly.

13. Lack of sun. The sun stimulates metabolism and alleviates depression and stress.

14. Nutritional deficiencies. Plain and simple, without proper nutrition metabolism will never be normal.

15. Heavy metal toxicity. Mercury from amalgam fillings can clog the liver and colon, and affect circulation.

18. Poor circulation. Clogged arteries cause poor circulation, which causes low metabolism.

19. Lack of oxygen. Most people have lower than normal levels of oxygen in their blood and cells. Sitting too long, not exercising causes this.

20. Allergies. Environmental and food allergies affect metabolism.

21. Parasites. Almost 100% of overweight people have parasites, usually stemming from having a clogged liver and colon.

22. Dieting. Every time you diet to lose weight your metabolism slows.

23. Lack of sweating. Sweating is a natural body process and a lack of sweating leads to a clogged lymphatic system and slower metabolism.

24. Low muscle mass. If your body does not have normal amounts of muscle your metabolism will be lower than normal.

25. Air conditioning. Research shows that exposure to the cold stimulates the appetite.

26. Eating no breakfast. People who skip breakfast eat almost twice as many calories during the rest of the day than people who eat a healthy breakfast.

27. EMS. Electromagnetic frequencies are generated from all wireless devices and have an adverse affect on every cell in the body, lowering the metabolic rate.

28. Eating before bed. Eating highly refined, or super highly refined foods, before bed causes low metabolism.

29. Genetically modified food. The body reacts to GMF in a way that lowers metabolism. In the United States almost all foods are genetically modified in some way.

30. Food additives. If food is not 100% organic then it is loaded with herbicides, pesticides, chemical fertilizers, antibiotics, and thousands of other man-made chemicals. American-produced food 100% will slow your metabolism unless it's organic.

31. Lack of walking. A lack of physical movement results in a constant lowering of the metabolic rate. Americans walk considerably less per day than people in other countries.

32. Antibiotics. Antibiotics kill germs and bad bacteria, but they also kill good bacteria.

From birth, microbes colonize us. After birth, while our immune systems are still undeveloped, these microbes learn to tolerate or destroy foreign substances. In order to develop a properly functioning immune system we must be exposed to a wide range of harmless microbes early in life. Unlike just a few generations ago we are exposed to antibiotics from birth. If the immune system is not familiar with external micros, it attacks them, which results in allergies and asthma. When the immune system turns on the body itself many other autoimmune diseases are seen. Minimizing immunization and exposing young children to a wide range of harmless germs is actually better for them than trying to overprotect them.

Resetting Your Metabolic Rate

1. Drink more water. Overweight people are almost always dehydrated. Drinking one large glass of water upon awakening is a great habit to start. You should be consuming close to one gallon of water throughout the day. Spring water is best but when it is not available drink water

that has been filtered by reverse osmosis if that isn't available drink distilled water. We suggest that people opt not to drink tap water because of all the chlorine, fluoride, and other contaminates found in it.

2. Insulin. Most overweight people are either pre-diabetic or already have diabetes. In people with diabetes the pancreas secretes insulin abnormally. If corrected a person can lose weight much easier and won't have to fight hunger while doing so. Three or four cups of coffee (or doses of caffeine) a day, helps keep blood sugar balanced. In fact, if you must have a sweet, always have it with a cup of coffee, or caffeine tablet.

3. Drink Coffee. In the amounts and at the times laid out for you in this book.

4. Whole Food Supplement. Each day take a whole food supplement which will provide your body with the needed nutrients.

5. Eating organic apples and grapefruit. Simply eating two organic apples and two organic grapefruits a day will regulate blood sugar, reduce appetite, and help to clean the liver, gallbladder and colon.

6. Eat Hot Peppers. Organic hot peppers and hot salsa stimulate an increase in metabolism and reduce appetite. Use organic hot salsa and organic hot peppers liberally as often as possible.

7. Eat Breakfast. Eating a large breakfast will reset the body's weight set point. We recommend eating a large breakfast that consists primarily of protein in the form of non-fat cottage cheese, plain, unsweetened yogurt, soy, free-ranging eggs, free ranging turkey, chicken, pork, and beef. 2/3 protein, 1/3 complex carbs. We suggest using organic raw butter or organic raw extra virgin olive oil as well.

8. Eat Six Times Per Day. It is important to eat more than just three meals a day. We suggest eating six times a day to reset your metabolism high so it will release abnormal fat reserves. It is best to eat a large breakfast followed by a mid-morning snack. After each meal have a snack that consists of organic fruits and vegetables. Remember, even if you don't feel hungry, eating at least six times a day will prove helpful in your goal of losing weight and becoming healthier.

9. Eat Dinner Before 6:00 p.m. Ideally, you should finish eating your dinner three and one-half hours before you go to bed. This is very important in resetting the hypothalamus so as not to store fat.

10. Eat Protein Before Bed. Eating 100 grams of organic beef, veal, chicken, turkey, or fish right before bedtime will stimulate the mobilization of fat cells as well as decrease water retention. This means you are burning fat while you sleep.

11. Eat Only Organic Meat And Dairy. Beef, chicken, turkey, milk, cheese, and all dairy products that are not certified organic are loaded with growth hormones, antibiotics, and other drugs. These products lead to obesity. Eating these products will create hormonal imbalances in the body leading to weight gain, abnormal storing of fat, menstrual cycle problems with women, PMS, and depression.

12. Eat Salad With Lunch and Dinner. In addition to whatever you choose to eat for lunch and dinner, add a big salad. Eating raw organic vegetables before your meal stimulates digestion. It also adds important fiber, which regulates blood sugar and appetite. Doing this will help reset the body's weight set point, while adding vital enzymes and nutrients that stimulate the release of stored fat.

13. Eat 100% Organic Food. Ideally, all the food you buy and consume should be labeled 100% organic. This means the food has not been genetically modified and has little, if any, man-made chemicals, preservatives, flavor enhancers, herbicides, pesticides, growth hormone, antibiotics, or other drugs. One hundred percent organic means 100% organic.

14. Walk. Walking outside at a slow steady pace for one hour per day will reset the body's weight set point. It may be hard to do this on a daily basis, but if you do you will see profound long-term effects. It is better to walk outside as opposed to using a treadmill. Be sure to keep your pace steady but don't overexert yourself. For example you want to get your heart rate up but still be able to maintain a conversation with your walking partner. Even if you can't commit to an hour a day, any walking is better than no walking. Just keep in mind that your goal is to be fit and lean; by walking you are literally one step closer to achieving this goal.

15. A Versa Climber. Exercise in any form is beneficial. A simple and easy exercise is a versa climber. It works both the upper and lower body at the same time. It releases beneficial endorphins and other hormones, and is the only exercise in the world that actually stimulates and exercises every cell in the body simultaneously. A Versa Climber improves muscle tone, muscle strength, flexibility, oxygenates the blood, improves circulation, and stimulates the release of toxins. Set it up in front of your television. Twenty to thirty minutes, once or twice a day, will have almost miraculous physical and mental health benefits.

16. Lift Weights. Doing any kind of resistance training, such as weight lifting, or using the machines available at exercise studios, is encouraged and beneficial. It will increase muscle mass, which will increase long-term improvement in the metabolism. Resistance training also releases hormones in the body that have anti-aging benefits, including improved skin and a youthful appearance. Strength increases, which leads to increased energy and vitality.

17. Yoga. Yoga can be done by any person no matter what your flexibility or physical condition. Yoga stimulates all the internal organs and promotes internal health. It increases flexibility and blood flow through the body. It strengthens and tones the muscles; it improves posture. It also unblocks the energy meridians through the body, dramatically increasing physical energy and emotional well-being.

18. No Trans Fats! Man-made trans fats absolutely, 100% of the time, will make you obese. They also lead to heart disease, cancer, arthritis, and diabetes. The most common trans fat is hydrogenated or partially hydrogenated oil of any kind. You cannot eat food with trans fats

19. No High Fructose Corn Syrup. If the food label says high fructose corn syrup, corn syrup, sucrose, dextrose, or malto dextrose, do not eat it. These man-made super high processed sugars have been designed to overtax the hypothalamus and make you fat.

20. No Artificial Sweeteners. Do not consume any food that has NutraSweet, Splenda, aspartame, sucralose, or saccharin on the label. These artificial sweeteners all adversely affect the hypothalamus and create the conditions for obesity. These artificial sweeteners are also highly chemically addicting and cause depression and anxiety.

21. No Monosodium Glutamate (MSG). MSG is a flavor enhancer and preservative. It is called an excitotoxin. It adversely affects the hypothalamus, as well as being chemically addicting. It will make you fat and leads to depression. Read the labels.

22. No Nitrites. Read the labels. If nitrites are listed, do not buy the product. Nitrites cause hormonal imbalances and will lead to weight gain, allergies, and food cravings.

23. No Farm Raised Fish. Farm raised fish live in cesspools of poison water. They are fed massive amounts of drugs and chemicals to increase growth and production. Much of the fish are injected with chemical food dyes to make them appear fresher longer. The chemicals and poisons found in these fish cause hormonal imbalances leading to weight gain and depression.

24. No Microwaving. Throw your microwave oven away. Any food that has been microwaved has been chemically altered into an unnatural state. Research shows eating any food that has been microwaved adversely affects blood cell counts and is linked to depression.

25. No Lotions or Creams. Look at all the products that you put on your skin. These include lotions, creams, soap, moisturizers, shampoos, bath gels, etc. People fifty years ago did not put

these types of products on their skin. Remember, the skin is the largest organ in the body. Whatever you put on your skin is absorbed into the bloodstream. When you put toxic, poisonous chemicals on your skin, they enter the bloodstream and adversely affect the organs and glands. The three most deadly ingredients you should avoid are mineral oil, propylene glycol, and sodium laureth sulfate. These are all poisons. Read the labels on the products you currently have. It is advised from here on you choose 100% organic products. Many doctors around the world believe that for good health if you can't eat it, don't put it on your skin!

26. No Fast Food. All fast food restaurants, as well as national and regional chains, should be avoided. The foods served are loaded with all of the ingredients that I mentioned above that should be avoided.

27. Drugs. Stop using all non-prescription, over-the-counter, and prescription drugs and medications of every kind absolutely. Of course you should first consult with your doctor. But it is important for you to know that they are proven to lead to weight gain and obesity. All non-prescription, over-the-counter, and prescription medications and drugs absolutely, 100%, cause illness and disease. The drug manufacturers themselves state this in their own printed literature. It is advised, only under the supervision of a licensed health care practitioner, that you avoid any and all non-prescription, over-the-counter medications, and prescription drugs. There are many all-natural non-drug alternatives that are proven to work better and have no negative side effects, but rather only health benefits. In 1950, less than 5% of the population took any kind of drug or medication on a regular basis. Today, it's an astonishing 70% of Americans who take medication or drugs on a regular basis.

28. Eliminate / Reduce Candida Yeast Overgrowth. Candida is a major cause of poor digestion. It is responsible for causing gas, bloating and constipation as well as many other unpleasant conditions. In order to eliminate food cravings you must avoid or reduce use of Candid Yeast Overgrowth.

29. Limit Carbonated Drinks. Carbonated drinks block calcium absorption and lead to nutritional deficiencies. They adversely affect digestion and the pancreas. They clog the liver and lymphatic system. These should be avoided. Try to choose a 100% organic non-carbonated beverage. It is far better to drink water, tea, freshly made juice, or coffee.

30. Reduce Air Conditioning. This is a mystery. Researcher have shown that people who spend long hours in air conditioning gain weight faster than those who don't. There are many theories to why this is true. I would encourage you to limit or reduce the amount of air conditioning you are exposed to.

31. Take Acetyl L-Carnitine. This amino acid helps turn fat into fuel. It also speeds the burning of fat cells and increasing metabolic rate.

32. Coral Calcium. Calcium supplementation has been shown to have major health benefits and increase weight loss. We suggest using a coral calcium which can be added to water.

33. Probiotics. Probiotics are friendly bacteria that when reintroduced into the body stimulate metabolism and improve digestion.

34. Using extra virgin raw coconut oil. This product is in most grocery stores. We recommend this type of oil because it stimulates metabolism and helps to improve digestion. It is also known to stimulate the thyroid.

35. Use raw organic apple cider vinegar. Using one tablespoon three times a day stimulates the metabolism and cleansing vital organs. It also releases stored fat cells.

36. Use Natural Sweeteners. If you need to use a sweetener, choose Naturolose as your first option. This is an all-natural herb which helps regulate blood sugar and stimulate weight loss. Other good options include raw organic agave nectar, raw organic honey, or raw organic sugar cane. Natural sweeteners are always better than artificial, chemically made sweeteners.

37. Use Cinnamon. Cinnamon helps regulate insulin and blood sugar. This helps

stimulate the hypothalamus into being reset to a normal state. Cinnamon normalizes appetite and helps release fat reserves.

38. Infrared Saunas. Sweating in a sauna increases metabolism and stimulates the release of fat cells. The skin is the largest organ in the body. Sweating in the sauna helps stimulates the release of accumulated toxins, increasing metabolism, bettering overall health, reducing appetite, and increasing metabolic rate. The two basic types of saunas are conventional saunas and infrared saunas with the infrared being the better choice.

39. Get Sun. Lack of sunlight on the body has been shown to lead to depression, overeating, increase in appetite, low metabolism, and weight gain. Ideally, twenty minutes in the sun over a naked body each day is recommended. Exposure to the sun increases the release of endorphins, eliminating depression and suppressing appetite. The sun is also the best source of Vitamin D, thus has been shown to prevent cancer.

40. Get Some Sleep. Researchers have concluded that lack of proper sleep leads to obesity. Ideally, you should go to bed at 10:00 p.m. and arise at 6:00 a.m. This is ideal. Getting eight hours of sleep is best. The body releases certain healing hormones between 11:00 p.m. and 2:00 a.m. Being in a deep sleep during this time promotes healing in the body, longevity, youthful appearance, eliminates depression, and helps the hypothalamus to stay in a state of operating norm

41. Colon Cleanse. We also recommend using colon cleansers every two months for the first year. Your skin, hair, and nails will look radiant and younger. This will help to balance any imbalances in your hormones and help you to lose more weight.

42. Colonics: We promise that it is well worth the cost to go and see a licensed colon therapist. For the first year go once a month to have a colonic and then once every three months following the first year. Cleaning the colon is absolutely necessary for weight loss and good health. A dramatic flattening of the stomach is noticed by people who do this on a routine basis. Most people lose an additional five to twenty pounds of excess weight. There are other benefits as well, such as reduced food cravings, gas, bloating, and constipation. In addition, having a clean colon means your body is absorbing nutrients more; this allows for increased energy and a general overall improvement of health.

43. Krill Oil. This oil comes from marine animals in Arctic waters. It has one of the highest concentrations of omega-3s. Taking this supplement increases circulation, increases oxygenation in the body, and promotes normal hormone levels. It has been shown to alleviate depression, decrease appetite, and is beneficial to the liver and pancreas. It is a tremendous aid to longevity and health as well as weight loss.

43. Vitamin E. All-natural Vitamin E promotes proper circulation, has heart healthy

benefits, and improves liver and gallbladder function. It is a powerful aid in weight loss, as well as promoting beautiful young-looking skin, and keeping your arteries open.

44. Digestive Enzymes. People who are overweight lack the ability to produce enough enzymes to digest food properly. To help bring the body back to normal you should take digestive enzymes with each meal.

45. Massage. Getting as many massages as possible, as often as possible, is highly encouraged. Vary the type of massage you receive. Massage will get everything moving in the body and speedup the weight loss process.

46. Shower Filter. Remember, your skin is the largest organ in the body. The water your shower in is loaded with fluoride, chlorine, and hundreds of other contaminants. Research has proven that when you take a shower your body absorbs more toxins than if you drank eight glasses of the same water. Getting a shower filter will allow you to bathe and shower in pure, fresh water.

Dry skin caused by the chlorine will disappear.

47. Heavy Metal Cleanse. To rid the body of heavy metals use a Chelation Complex product. This will improve circulation. It will also increase energy and metabolism.

48. Electromagnetic Chaos Eliminator. We are bombarded by invisible electromagnetic energy every day. This did not exist fifty years ago. Today, however, with satellites, radio transmissions, cell phones, wireless devices, high-definition TVs, and an array of electronic products, every cell in our body is being smashed with trillions of bits of unnatural electromagnetic chaos. Researchers have now proven that this adversely affects the cells in our body. Use of electromagnetic chaos eliminators will lead to increased energy, better mental clarity, better body function and reducing of depression.

49. Breathe. Interestingly enough, the majority of people in America do not breathe fully and deeply, thus have a body that is deficient in oxygen. Research has shown that if overweight people did nothing else but deep breathing for ten minutes, two times a day, they would still lose weight. You can do this while driving in your car, watching TV, or sitting in front of your computer. For specific breathing techniques and methods, review my book, "The Perfect Day."

50. Fluorescent Lights. Being exposed to florescent lights should be avoided or eliminated. Florescent lighting causes chemical reactions in the brain that product fatigue and depression. This leads to food cravings. Florescent lighting also negatively affects the cells of the body, suppressing the immune system and lowering the metabolism.

51. De-stressing CDs. I cannot emphasize how important stress reduction is in reducing hunger, increasing metabolism, alleviating depression, and promoting long-term permanent weight loss. Listening to a stress reducing CD once per day has profound emotional, mental, and health benefits.

52. Add Fiber. Adding fiber to your diet will help speed up the weight loss process dramatically. It will reduce appetite, relieve constipation, improve digestion, and help cleanse the body of toxins, help increase energy, and help correct years of eating super highly refined food.

53. Parasites. Eliminating parasites is important for weight loss. Virtually everyone has parasites that are partially responsible for a host of medical symptoms including inability to lose weight. These are also responsible for food and environmental allergies, asthma, skin disorders, constipation, gas and bloating, and can lead to ulcers, diabetes, and even cancer. Do a complete parasite cleanse.

54. Liver Cleanse. In virtually all obese people tested, a clogged or sluggish liver exists. This leads to improper metabolism of fat, slowing of digestion, increased appetite, low metabolism, and is partially responsible for food cravings. When the liver is cleansed and operating properly, every organ and gland in the body can work more efficiently. This increases energy, decreases depression, increases metabolism, lowers hunger, and dramatically increases an overall sense of wellbeing.

Some Good News

There are many factors we deal with every day that keep our metabolism low. Believe it or not the above list is only some of them. The list may seem overwhelming, but it is just the beginning. These factors hold overweight people prisoner because they keep the metabolism so low you are guaranteed to keep gaining weight. You are also guaranteed to fail at losing weight by using any of the conventional methods.

We have discussed all the bad things that occur when you have a low metabolism. Let us take a look at the positive things that occur when your metabolic rate is brought back to normal. The first thing you will notice is a dramatic increase in energy. You will feel more motivated. You will notice an improvement in your skin, hair, and even your nails. As you have a stronger immune system you will find that your entire body is functioning better. There is evidence that suggests once the metabolism is corrected a person's lifespan increases.

One primary cause of intense and constant hunger is food manufacturers who are intentionally creating food using food additives and chemicals that are specifically designed to affect the hypothalamus in a manner which increases hunger. Food manufacturers, like pharmaceutical companies, are developing products with the intention of creating a physical, chemical addiction to the food. There is overwhelming evidence that the chemicals used in making and cooking of fast food and processed foods increases hunger and lowers metabolism.

As we touched on earlier, the motive for those in the food industry is profit. The only way that will happen is to get more people to buy and eat more food. Publicly traded food companies are producing genetically modified food using chemical poison fertilizers, herbicides and pesticides.

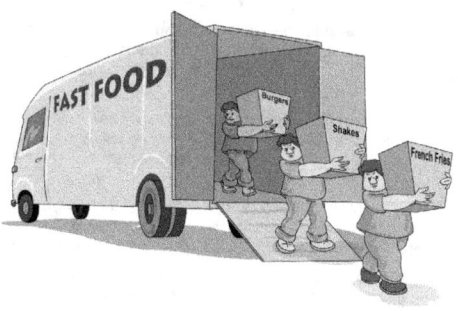

Food is ripened with poisonous gas, injected with chemical preservatives and flavoring agents. Food is eradiated, pasteurized and bathed in poisonous chlorine baths. Then it is injected with antibiotics and growth hormones. Food is produced in an unnatural, abnormal way. Even fruits and vegetables are affected. All commercially produced fruits, vegetables, meat, dairy, poultry and fish are laced with thousands of man-made chemicals hormones, and drugs.

The greatest cause of obesity today is that in America the food supply is being purposely produced to increase food cravings, create intense hunger and bingeing. Most bread made in the United States is extremely fattening; this is not so in other countries. Likewise, other products such as; milk, butter, and cheese made in America are also extremely fattening, but not so in other countries. Many times, when foreigners visit the United States they gain weight because even though they are eating similar foods they are not the same at all.

It is the man-made chemicals in food that really make a person overweight. That is why being busy counting calories and carbohydrates or needlessly worrying about the fat and protein in the food you eat does not work unless these other issues are addressed first.

A Healthy Agenda vs. Food Companies' Agenda

Another problem is that when many people consume small amounts of food throughout the day that are high on the glycemic index, the hypothalamus gets shocked. When this happens, the body abnormally stores fat and the metabolism rises for a little while, the drops for a long while. Many people skip breakfast and even lunch only to have a large meal later in the day. This is the exact scenario in which the hypothalamus will be shocked.

The good news is there is a simple solution, and that is the Caffeine Diet. It will protect you from food companies. You will even be able to ignore the television ads for food that are designed to make you crave food like a dog in a Pavlovian experiment. As part of the Caffeine Diet you will no longer be a slave to the food companies.

Food companies spend billions of dollars in advertising in magazines, newspapers, and on television and radio networks. These media outlets are controlled by the agenda and revenues of the advertisers.

This book will be an instant enemy of the food industry. We want people to be cured of their obesity, food cravings, low metabolism, and intense hunger; that means you will be eating and buying less food.

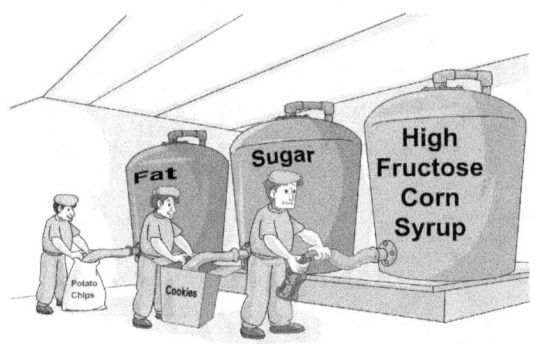

You can compare today's food industry with the tobacco industry. They knew that smoking cigarettes caused cancer and other diseases but due to pure greed they lied about it for fifty years. This resulted in tens of thousands of deaths every year. The current food producers know that their genetically-modified, chemically-laced food products cause obesity, and they know that due to those chemicals, people will always choose food based on taste, rather than what is healthy.

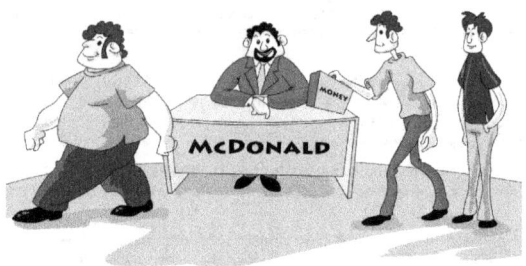

In other parts of the world people are not counting carbs or calories. They are paying no attention to how much salt or sugar is in the food they eat. They drink beer, eat bread with every meal and have ice cream before bed. They are eating real food-real, full fat milk, cheese, and butter as well as chicken and other poultry with the skin on. They don't even make light beer in most other countries. So why are people thin in these other countries? The answer is quite simple. The food is produced naturally, with no genetically modified chemicals or additives that trigger the appetite and binge eating.

It's not that beef makes you fat; it's the chemicals and growth hormones and drugs put in the American beef that makes you fat. It's not the bread in America but all the added high fructose corn syrup and other man-made sweeteners, all of which lower metabolism and increase appetite. Again let me make it clear to you: the American food supply is being produced with the purpose of making you fat.

Prepackaged diet foods are loaded with monosodium glutamate, high fructose corn syrup, and thousands of man-made chemicals. You may lose some weight initially, but you will not lose it in the areas you want to lose it, and you will not reshape your body. You will, however, lower your metabolism and increase your hunger. This ensures that once you stop dieting you will immediately gain all the weight back, plus more.

In the movie documentary, *Super Size Me,* Morgan Spurlock ate only at McDonalds for one month. He gained twenty-eight pounds in that time. McDonald's food is specifically designed to trigger your appetite and make you a slave to that type of food.

There are more than 2000 calories in the typical fast food meal, along with massive amounts of man-made trans fats. You will also find in every meal high fructose corn syrup and artificial sweeteners. These chemicals will cause you to have an abnormally operating hypothalamus, which as we know ensures you will become overweight and stay that way. The more overweight a person is the more food they will eat, and this means lots of money for companies like McDonalds.

On the Caffeine Diet your body shape will change dramatically. The fat on the hips, thighs, buttocks, belly, and breast will really seem to vanish. Fat deposits will be used as fuel, which will increase energy. You will also notice a decrease in appetite and how much food you eat. As your health improves so will your disposition.

When you are losing weight every day you will be highly motivated to continue on with the program. Another benefit is that on the Caffeine Diet hunger almost vanishes. Unlike other programs, on this diet you will have more energy, and feel more positive, with no food cravings at all.

You will lose inch after inch as your stomach gets flat and your waist gets smaller. The before and after photos of people who have done this protocol are amazing. Many people have had friends or family ask if they have had liposuction.

With most other weight loss methods, time-consuming exercise is almost always required. We strongly encourage exercise but it is not required to produce the results we constantly see. In fact, we have purposely had clients do no exercise at all to make sure these spectacular results could be achieved without exercise and they had great success.

One of the most exciting things that people experience is a fast and dramatic flattening of the stomach. When you look in the mirror and like what you see, and also get on the scale and like the number you see, it is extremely motivating.

As long as you are on the Caffeine Diet you will be able to eat like a normal weight person and burn calories like a normal weight person. Once your hunger and appetite mechanisms are rebalanced you won't suffer with physiological food cravings. This means that you will have no desire to eat when you are not hungry, and for many people this alone is a life-changing experience.

Imagine not having to deal with willpower or the feeling you are depriving yourself of something you want. Imagine not being hungry and no longer being a slave to food or your appetite. The Caffeine Diet may truly be the answer to your prayers.

CHAPTER THIRTEEN –A CLOSER LOOK AT CAFFEINE AND EXERCISE

I didn't run out of energy, I ran till I ran out of coffee – Dr. Jeffry Weiss

Caffeine and Exercise: Good or Bad for Your Cardiovascular System?

Several studies have suggested that, in a healthy person, caffeine can actually improve the way the heart responds to exercise. For example, a 1995 study of caffeine found that, in patients with normal blood pressure, a dose of caffeine can *help* the heart handle exercise by slowing the heart rate, reduce blood pressure, and thus ease the work load on the heart.

If these results seem surprising or even paradoxical to you, you are not alone. The lead researcher commented that, "The outcomes of the study were a surprise to me. We would have thought the opposite would be true." Although his conclusions were based on observations of lowered blood pressure and increased heart output in six healthy young men, he asserted that it was plausible to imagine that people with heart disease (but without arrhythmia) could also benefit from an amount of caffeine equivalent to two cups of coffee. If this is so, it contradicts the conventional medical wisdom that has prompted doctors to routinely advise patients with heart problems to stop drinking coffee.

Another exercise benefit for some heart patients was asserted in a 1984 study that claimed caffeine was a "booster of pain-free walking time for patients with chronic stable angina." This study found that drinking a couple of cups of coffee a day increased the time such patients could exercise by as much as 12 percent, while decaffeinated coffee had no effect.

Caffeine and Exercise: a Good Combination?

There is conflicting evidence when it comes to determining whether caffeine has a positive or negative effect on people exercising. There are studies that suggest caffeine improves how the heart functions during exercise. People with no known heart conditions have been found to show a slower heart rate and lower blood pressure when they add caffeine to their normal exercise routine. This study also showed that people who already have heart disease can benefit from a small amount of caffeine. This of course contradicts what most doctors recommend. Caffeine has been found to relieve pain for people suffering from angina. These individuals were able to exercise for considerably longer periods of time when drinking caffeinated coffee as opposed to decaffeinated.

Caffeine: a Performance Enhancer

Many exercise enthusiast and professional athletes will tell you that caffeine helps to improve performance. It is especially helpful when endurance and speed are important as caffeine enhances both. Long distance cyclists, runners, and cross country skiers have used caffeine to improve performance. There are reports that even race horses are now being tested for the use of caffeine.

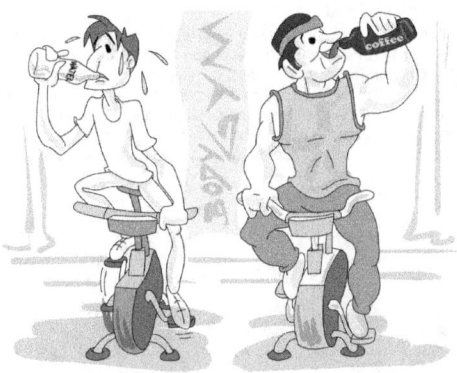

How Caffeine Affects the Body During Exercise

A study conducted in the later part of the 1990s found that 200 mg. of caffeine had significant impact on endurance. There are many other studies since then that have found this to be true. In order to understand how caffeine improves aerobic performance, we will review some of those studies and conclusions.

There are a few ways in which the body gets the energy needed to power muscles, dependent on whether the energy expenditure is short, moderate, or extended. Energy also burns differently in different muscles depending on their size.

Athletes burn energy differently than people who are out of shape. There are other variables to consider as well. We need to look at caffeine dose, pre-exercise food consumption, and individual variations in response to tolerance. These many variables may explain why the findings from research are sometimes inconsistent.

There are three assertions that affect how the basic theory on caffeine and athletic performance is seen. First we look at the question as to what degree caffeine increases the efficiency with which the body burns fat. Caffeine increases free fatty acid mobilization. This process delays the depletion of glycogen by encouraging the muscles to use fat as fuel. This delays exhaustion. In high-intensity exercise this is crucial. In lower intensity exercise the effects are not seen as dramatically.

Next we must look at the way in which caffeine enhances the efficiency of burning sugars. This is especially important because glycogen is a primary source of energy for exercise. Exhaustion occurs once glycogen has been lost. During the first minutes of exercise the effect of the glycogen-sparing can best be observed. This is due to the fact that during the first 15-20 minutes of exercise the body uses almost 50 percent of the glycogen. When the glycogen is spared it can be utilized later in the exercise routine.

Last we observe how caffeine can lower the rate of perceived exertion (RPE) reducing our sense of fatigue. Studies report athletes show significantly less exertion during exercise after consuming caffeine.

Caffeine: how much of an advantage?

Let's face it, most athletes are looking for any legal way of having an advantage over the competition. This may be one reason why the use of sports snacks is increasing among athletes and weekend warriors. Only performance boosters containing carbohydrates or caffeine have been endorsed for use by the United States Armed Forces. There are obviously other ingredients that benefit users but there hasn't been enough research to date to confirm such findings. However there has been research done which shows that consumption of about 900 mg. of caffeine (3 large cups of coffee) can increase endurance time from thirty to fifty minutes.

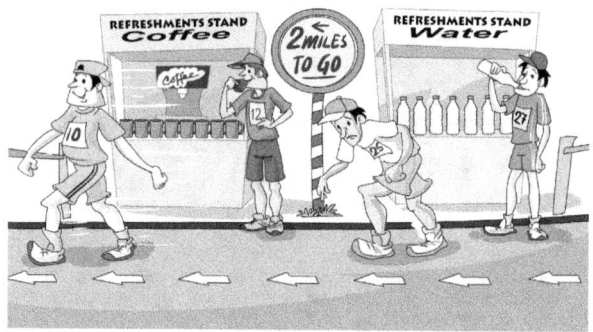

One study found that if caffeine was consumed one hour before weight lifting users were able to increase the amount of reps they did. They were also able to bench press approximately five more pounds than when they didn't use caffeine prior to working out.

This study also concluded that caffeine reduced muscle pain and allowed the athletes to work out longer than they could otherwise.

There haven't been enough studies on how caffeine affects other ordinary activities like walking. Experiments still need to be done on this subject. The effects of caffeine as an athletic performance-booster are better understood when it comes to more intense exercise as we have previously discussed.

Caffeine and the Weekend Athlete

Athletes who train and exercise on a regular basis have more effective antioxidant defenses. They are better tuned. Weekend athletes are considered to be people that usually don't exercise during the week but usually just on the weekends. This group of athletes is in a special predicament. They are more open to damage muscles because they aren't exercising consistently. Caffeine is especially important for people who aren't training regularly because it speeds muscle recovery time and healing. Caffeine can also effectively make up for the weaker defense system against free radicals found in the weekend athletes. Caffeine accomplishes this by delivering a powerful antioxidant when it is most needed. Caffeine reduces sensitivity to pain. This reduction of pain means people can work out harder and for longer periods of time. Caffeine triggers the release of epinephrine from the adrenal glands, which improves muscle contractions. A person experiences a reduction in perceived exertion that allows them to push more weight with less perceived exertion. A person can experience increased muscle mass if they use caffeine regularly before exercising.

When And How Much To Take

It is hard to determine exactly when the caffeine should be taken. There is question concerning which method of administration is more effective as well. The reality is that even if there are parameters as to how much and when most people should take caffeine in relation to exercise, each person would still need to find out for themselves through experimentation.

There are many scientific studies that don't consider the varying weights of test subjects. If a dosage given doesn't take into consideration a person's size, the effects can be very misleading. Also, most studies are done taking a single dose of caffeine before exercising. There have been only a few done considering the effects of repeated doses before and during exercise.

Research has shown that ingesting around 300 mg. of caffeine can improve endurance by 25%. For our purposes, we suggest taking caffeine 30-45 minutes before exercise, then working out for 60-90 minutes. A post-workout meal is beneficial and your appetite should be recovered by that time. The suggested dosage is 2 mg. per pound of bodyweight. For example: 150 pound person = 300 mg. of caffeine. The following pages provide more specific guidelines for using caffeine to achieve your personal goals, and maximize your athletic performance.

Timing

We know caffeine is rapidly absorbed by the body, with the highest blood levels of the drug achieved within one hour. During the first 15 minutes 75% of the benefits are received. In most studies exercise is not performed until an hour after consuming caffeine. It is important to note here the half-life of 100 mg. of caffeine averages between 2 and 3 hours. This tells us that caffeine is excreted by the body relatively slowly. Many people maintain blood concentrations close to the maximum level for approximately 2 hours. It takes most people around 15-20 minutes to feel a significant effect. It takes another 15 minutes to an hour for the peak effects to kick in.

Researchers are still unsure if the fat burning effect of caffeine contributes to the athletic enhancement. The fat burning effect occurs about 3 hours after taking caffeine. Due to the many variables that encompass each individual, average values fail to give an accurate guide.

It is best for the individual to experiment using caffeine at different intervals before exercising. Experimenting will provide you with an accurate timetable so you can get the maximizing ergogenic effect from caffeine.

Factors that Influence the Half Life of Caffeine

There are three main factors that influence how long caffeine will remain in the body. The half-life is the length of time needed for the body to rid itself of ½ of a chemical substance.

1) Smoking, Oral Contraceptives, and drinking grapefruit juice: All of these actions work to shorten the half-life of caffeine.

2) Genetic predisposition: The half-life of caffeine is different from individual to individual due to metabolic factors that are determined by genetics.

3) The amount of caffeine ingested taken: If you took 200 mg. in an hour you'll be feeling the

effects less than you would if you had taken 400 mg. of caffeine. Another way of looking at this is if you took 300 mgs., you would most likely feel the effects for around 4-5 hours. If you double that dose to 600 you will feel the significant for 6-7 hours. These amounts are different from person to person dependent of body mass and genetic factors.

The More You Do for You, the More Caffeine Will Do for You

Studies have shown that trained athletes get more positive, predictable results from using caffeine than the average person does. One study showed an Olympic athlete improved his endurance by over half an hour using caffeine. Caffeine has a direct action on muscle tissue; and the muscles of highly trained athletes are obviously different than those of the average person. This difference might explain why the highly trained athlete is more responsive to caffeine's effects.

We have already looked at how caffeine affects performance with the way it increases stamina and provides more resistance to pain. Using caffeine alone is comparable to taking an ibuprofen. We have also learned that in many experiments caffeine increases the power of painkillers and other nonsteroidal anti-inflammatory drugs (NSAIDs).

Caffeine and Attitude

The phrase "having a winning attitude" refers to when an athlete believes that they will succeed often times they do. Caffeine works to create a more optimistic attitude in people and this ability to lift spirits and morale also benefit athletes. It's difficult to quantify benefits like these that are a combination of pain relief and an attitude adjuster. But there is no doubt that caffeine helps people become and stay winners.

Caffeine vs. Amphetamines

Caffeine, when used beyond reasonable amounts, creates unpleasant side effects like jitteri-ness, irritability, and insomnia. When you take more caffeine than the standards recommended it actually does less of what you want and more of what you don't want. Most people find what works for them and they stick with that throughout their lifetime without any significant change.

With amphetamines people have a strong and often time's irresistible craving to consume more, and because people build a tolerance to these drugs, higher dose are constantly needed. There is also no need to increase your caffeine intake as there appears to be no tolerance build up when it comes to the ergogenic effects.

The most profound difference is an obvious one. Other drugs cause all kinds of very negative side effects. They cause mental, emotional, and physical problems. People end up in jails and institutions because of unregulated amphetamine use. This cannot be said of coffee. Caffeine is a regular part of most people's lives and never causes any of these types of problems.

Caffeine and Dehydration

This is one of the prime myths we addressed earlier. We know of no published study that has shown caffeine to have any detrimental effects on athletic performance when taken in moderation. Athletes are cautioned when it comes to caffeine as it is feared to be a diuretic. There is no proof at all that caffeine will dehydrate athletes. One study found that caffeine ingestion during rest causes a very mild increase in urinary output; however caffeine ingestion with exercise produced no diuretic effect. There were no changes found in fluid or electrolyte balance. In other words caffeine's diuretic effect seems to affect a person who is not exercising in ways that it doesn't affect a person who is exercising.

Self Assessment and Your Caffeine Intake

There are no average test scores given here. The tests that follow are to help you to see how caffeine can improve your athletic performance. This will enable you set goals for yourself and experiment with caffeine to find the best amounts for you.

To start, we suggest a person weighing 150 pounds uses 100 mg. of caffeine. We have listed corresponding dosages for people of different weights given in Appendix "H". It comes out to be approximately 2 mg. of caffeine per kilogram. You can increase your caffeine dosage gradually by 50 or 100 mg. if needed. Once you find the optimum dosage there is no need to continue increasing this amount.

Take your caffeine approximately one half hour before you begin testing and take it in a single dose. Once you've found your optimum dosage try dividing the dosage during the longer tests (1/2 dose at the beginning, then a half dose 1-2 hours later). Another experiment you may want to try is to take all of your caffeine 2-3 hours before you exercise to see if the increased burning of fat improves your performance.

Note: As always we highly suggest that you consult your doctor before embarking on these or any other tests of athletic capacity.

The Endurance Test

For this test you need to experiment to determine what you consider a normal speed for you when it comes to running or cycling. We suggest you experiment further to determine what "fast" is for you as well. Next you will want to try using different doses at different times throughout the day to see what effect, if any, these variables have on your performance. It is very important that you take notes during this process and see how long it takes for you to reach exhaustion during each experiment. Try the same techniques running at your normal pace and then at your predetermined fast pace and take note of any changes you see when you introduce caffeine into the equation. It is important that you are in good health and well rested when you are conducting your tests.

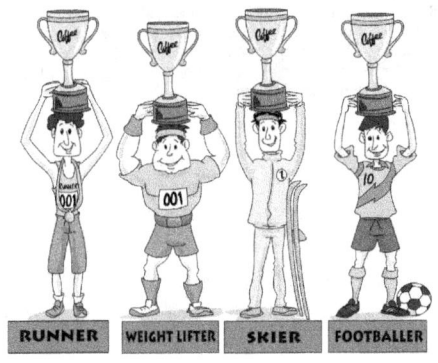

Caffeine and Weight Lifting

In this test you will be using several different weights. Have at least four different weights ranging from 2-20 lbs. Take note of how many repetitions you can complete when your body is caffeine free. Then take caffeine before (15 – 60 minutes) doing your repetitions and see if there is any change. Try the same approach we recommended for running and cycling. Take different amounts of caffeine at different times. Find what your average is without caffeine first, and then take note of any changes once caffeine is introduced.

The following test is only for experienced weight lifters who have a partner they are working out with. You will be using a barbell to determine the maximum weight you can lift with and without caffeine use. Again try different doses at different times and make note of any additional lifting power that caffeine gives you.

Reaction Time

Some of you may already have an awareness of how caffeine impacts your reaction time in certain sports like tennis that require a quick response. Still, you may benefit from taking the "Reaction Time" test because you may find that a higher dose can improve your reaction time further, or decrease it if a greater dose provides no additional benefit.

Recommended Exercise Equipment

Now, what if there was a machine that you could work out with within the confines of your own home, that would burn three times as many calories as walking, that you could watch TV while using, that wouldn't require a trainer, special workout clothes, or traveling to a gym where you would be uncomfortable and stand out, and cost less than $1000?* Would you be interested? Well it's true. This is not a miracle or a fantasy. It's a stair stepper. It's the only piece of equipment that uses both upper and lower body muscles at the same time where you can adjust the tension and requires only three square feet of floor space. It will fit in even the smallest apartment. And you'll never even miss your favorite sit-com. Yes, TV is actually good for something. By distracting you, you will work out longer, with more intensity than if you were just focused on the workout (pick comedies because laughter triggers the release of endorphins that will enable you to work out longer). For those more adventuresome, there are other exercise routines that do not require going to the gym, but that can be just as effective. I call these "Urban Exercises." See Appendix "A" for a detailed list of urban exercises, gym-based exercises, free weight and machine workouts, and home alternatives.

*Base on current e-bay prices.

CHAPTER FOURTEEN – BEYOND CAFFEINE: DIET AND NUTRITION

The discovery of coffee has enlarged the realm of possibility and given more promise to hope - Isidore Bourdon

What Nature Intended

What we eat is a function of who we are. Man is classified by science as a primate. The order Primata evolved from the order Insectivora, or insect-eating mammals. Ninety-five percent of primates have a single-chambered stomach incapable of digesting most complex carbohydrates as they occur in nature. Of the two hundred species of primates, only the Colobus and Langur monkeys have a multi-chambered stomach and are thus capable of digesting a diet consisting primarily of grains. Compared to other primates, man has a shrunken large intestine and colon. In evaluating the gut ratios (the size of the small intestine to the large intestine) ours is much less similar to other primates and more comparable to carnivores, specifically the wolves.

As explained by Ray Audette in his book *Neanderthin*, "our relatively small lower gastrointestinal tract inhibits our ability to extract nutrients from calorically sparse food such as leaves, shoots, grains, barks, etc., making us more dependent on calorically dense food such as meat, fish, fruit, and nuts."

As we evolved, our larger hominid brain required greater amounts of energy even as our digestive systems became smaller in relation to both brain size and total body size.

At this stage of evolution, man could no longer survive on the low-energy-value food favored by our early ancestors. Recent studies have shown that monkeys fail to thrive or reproduce when their diets do not include high quality protein. And modern vegetarians experience the same developmental problems as meat-starved monkeys.

One of the most essential vitamins is B^{12}. Our requirement for B^{12} can only be met by eating meat or fish, or by supplementation. And only fish and meat are packed with enough fats and calories to supply the necessary energy demanded by the brain of man. In fact, within a few hundred years after the inception of the agricultural revolution, and man's dependence on grains, his brain sized has decreased by 11%! It has only been in the past several thousand years that our brains returned to their pre-agrarian size.

Meat and fish are a better source of energy for the body than sugars. The fats in meat and fish provide energy by breaking down into glucose. The breakdown only occurs as needed, sparing the body the effects of high levels of blood sugar as well as the extreme swings in blood sugar levels we see when we eat sugar and simple carbohydrates.

Without the constant supply of energy from simple carbohydrates, the body will produce more of the enzymes needed to utilize fat as the primary source of energy. The body will thereby be spared the dangers of relying on sugars as the primary fuel and being constantly subjected to the insulin effect. (You can see why diabetes is becoming an epidemic in today's world by realizing that many people do exactly the opposite of these findings and conclusions).

Elizabeth Somer said, in her book, *Origin Diet*, "Our diets today are killing us because they are as alien to our bodies as breathing carbon monoxide." She goes on to say, "For 99% of the time humans have been on earth, they have eaten and evolved on diets of nuts, seeds, honey, plants, fish, and very lean wild game. Our ancestors not only survived on this diet, but lived virtually free of heart disease, cancer, diabetes, auto immune disorders, hypertension, osteoporosis, and other modern diseases."

Ms. Somer continues, "We may wear designer clothes, and live in air conditioned houses, but we are still genetically programmed to live and eat as we did since we climbed out of trees. Our biochemistry and physiology remain fine-tuned to the diets and activities and communality of our ancestors."

Outsmarted By Technology

The problem occurs when genetics clash with technology. In order to make certain that man maximized nutrient consumption at each meal, the brain and the stomach released biochemicals (endorphins, dopamine, serotonin) that stimulated the appetite and brought on a feeling of euphoria. Yet now, with food readily available, eating is a maladaptive response; technology has moved faster than genetics. We still have the biological systems of our ancestors from 6½ million years ago, but with the availability of all the food our supermarkets can hold.

Live to Eat Or Eat to Live?

At the core of all our actions is a central reward system. And that reward system is measured by endorphin release. Endorphins create euphoria and pain relief.

Endorphins are triggered by stimuli from our internal and external worlds, by our psychological desires or physiological actions.

One of the most important attributes of endorphins is their capacity to promote a sense of well-being. In fact, some endorphins are known to be hundreds of times stronger than opiates like morphine and heroin!

Enkephalins (short-lived endorphins triggered by the consumption of fat and sugary foods) stimulate the hypothalamus (the part of the brain that controls appetite) to continue eating. This system of reward overrides the signals from the stomach and intestines that would normally tell the brain to shut down the eating process.

We may believe that there is no connection between our day-to-day actions and decisions, and our feelings of contentment. Yet what we perceive as sudden, disconnected moments of euphoria are, in reality, very specific responses to chosen behaviors.

In 1993, an experiment was conducted to determine the power of endorphins. Scientists inserted electrodes into the brains of rats. The rats ran a maze, after which they could either pull a lever that would, through the electrodes, trigger the release of endorphins, or they could pull a lever that provided nutritious food or provide sex. The results were that the rats chose endorphins, neglecting sex and food, which, in some cases, resulted in death. And each day we humans run our own maze, fueled predominately by food, rewarded by endorphins and the euphoric feelings they provide.

Endorphins have four key roles. One, they reduce stress. Two, they relieve pain. Three, they strengthen the immune system. Four, they delay the aging process. And recently, scientists have discovered that endorphins can activate natural killer cells in our body, boosting the body's defenses against cancer. Endorphins also appear to affect mood, memory retention, and learning. And endorphins help us maintain our precarious emotional balance.

All things we choose, we do to maximize the flow of endorphins. We may think that it is external circumstances that make us happy or fulfilled or satiated, but it is really biochemical reactions in the body that set these feelings in motion.

How you can gain control our appetite by choosing the right foods and supplements, and engage in alternative behaviors that stimulate endorphin release is the key. And the key to that understanding is an appreciation of the five behaviors that trigger endorphin release. These are:

1 - Eating
2 - Exercise
3 – Shared Compassion, Love, Camaraderie
4 - Adaptation To New Situations
5 - Interaction With Enriched Environments

The joy we derive from a hug, a workout in the gym, a walk in nature, a good meal, taking on a new hobby, or sharing intimately with a friend or loved one are all produced by endorphins. And by engaging in alternative behaviors that stimulate endorphin release we can overcome our food dependency!

As man ate, powerful, addictive biochemicals (endorphins) were released into the bloodstream, reinforcing the most vital of human activities. The same feeling of satisfaction, even happiness, that we feel after a full meal (think Thanksgiving), our ancestors felt from a variety of sources - besides food - each and every day.

We took from them our endorphin set-point, but left behind socialization, nature, and the need for daily physical activity. We went from diversity and extended families to specialization and separation.

We live to eat. Our ancestors ate to live – subsisting on a diet of nuts, leaves, fruits, grasses, bugs, plants, lean wild game, and fish. They remained free of heart disease, cancer, diabetes, hypertension, osteoporosis, cataracts, and other modern diseases.

Now that you're on Caffeine Diet, and able to control our appetite and choose the foods best for your health, what's next? Let's start where we all start . . . . with breakfast. For those of you who do not currently eat breakfast, here's some interesting statistics for you:

1) Those who eat breakfast away from home have a 137% increased in the risk of becoming obese.

2) Those who did not eat breakfast at all had a 450% increased risk of becoming obese.

3) Those who did not eat breakfast had a higher body mass index (BMI), and had less energy during the day.

4) Those who ate breakfast were less inclined to snack compulsively than those who skipped breakfast.

5) Those who skipped breakfast wound up eating 40% more calories during the day.

6) Those who ate a protein-based breakfast - such as eggs, ham, cottage cheese, and yogurt - felt fuller longer, and consumed fewer calories for at least 24 hours afterwards. Two groups were compared. One group, that ate a bagel, jelly regular cereal, consumed a daily average of 2,035 calories. The protein-based group ate 1,761 calories.

How Much Should You Eat?

It is extremely difficult to eat too much if you are consuming natural, whole foods. It is only sugars - that stimulate the appetite, and provide empty calories - that do not fill you up, and that stimulate you (by an insulin reaction or endorphin release) to eat more than you should. Focusing

147

on calories is not necessarily beneficial. However, for those who feel the need for guidelines, consider the following to estimate your calorie needs:

1. Multiply your desired weight by ten calories per pound. For example, if you currently weigh 160 pounds, but know that 140 is your healthier weight: Multiply 140

pounds x ten calories per pound. The resulting calories are what you require to simply breathe, pump blood, and grow hair. It is called your resting metabolic rate (RMR).

2. Add to your RMR to account for your daily activities. If you are moderately active, add 50 percent of your RMR (1400 x 50%), or 700 calories. This brings your daily caloric needs to 1,400 + 700 = 2,100. For a sedentary profession, add zero; extremely active (load concrete bags), add 100%.

3. Now add additional calories for your "purposeful exercise program." That is, if you exercise aerobically for about 45 minutes, add 300 to 400 calories; if you run for three miles, add about 300 calories. This brings you to:

Resting metabolic rate	1,400
Daily activity	700
Purposeful exercise (free weights, etc)	300
Aerobics	400
Total calories/day required to maintain weight	2,800

What should you eat?

Paleolithic man had the lowest fat-to-total-body-weight ratio of any people on earth – even though they ate more than the average active American. They were amazingly fit and had powerful muscle tone. The men averaged 5'10", the women 5'8". Their physiology was the equivalent of elite athletes of today, and they evolved as such through the following regime:

Meat eating: The forces of natural selection molded and shaped our physiology to function optimally on a diet consisting primarily of meat. How can we be certain of the foods our ancestors ate? Archeological evidence shows that the teeth of our ancestors had a thin enamel coating. This implies that they ate a diet consisting mostly of softer foods. The teeth of mammals that subsisted on bark and fibrous plants show heavy wear. And tools found at archeological sites include fishhooks, axes, harpoons and other tools used to trap, kill, and skin game. All this evidence gives us a good idea of what they primarily ate.

Most experts agree that game hunting was the primary means of sustenance for millions of years, up to the beginnings of the agricultural revolution 10,000 years ago. It has been estimated by forensic pathologists that from 30 to 40% of the calories consumed by our ancestors were in the form of large and small wild game, fish, birds, eggs, reptiles, and insects.

Variety of foods: Pollen found at other sites confirmed that Paleolithic man grew and ate a variety of plants. Hair samples examined by researchers at the University of Virginia found that the diet of our ancestors varied greatly depending on the opportunities that hunting and foraging provided.

An analysis of the diets of modern-day hunter-gatherers - such as the IKung San of southern Africa and the Ache of Paraguay - confirm that the diets of most hunter-gatherers consist of a great variety of root crops, fruit, and free-ranging animals. We can, from these studies and comparisons, estimate that the diet of our ancestors consisted of 35% of calories from fish and lean game, 35% of calories from plants, seeds, nuts, and omega-3 fatty acids, and 30% from fruit and honey. Dr. S. Boyd Eaton has estimated that, on average, our highly active ancestors consumed 3,000 calories a day.

Conclusion: The foods our ancestors ate ensured longevity and the best chance to pass on their genes – as opposed to those provided by domestication or farming. We have, in a matter of a few thousands years, contradicted nature and natural selection, going from a diet that averaged 35% of calories from protein (fish, meat, poultry, nuts and seeds), to one where we now derive 17% of our calories from very poor sources of protein. As a species, we could very well naturally select ourselves right out of evolution. Remember, only the fittest survive. Now let's see how the diet of our ancestors compares with the recommendations made by those of us who have dedicated a lifetime to studying evolutionary biology and behavior.

What to Eat / What Not to Eat

Choosing what to eat must be a simple task, for if it is not, we will never maintain the regime. In fact, the rules are very simple:

Do Eat	Don't Eat
Berries	Sugar
Fruits (in moderation!)	Cakes, Pies, Doughnuts
Vegetables (darkest colors are best)	Potatoes (except yams and sweet)
Nut and Seeds (except peanuts)	Chocolate
Meat and poultry (organically grown -	White bread, processed
free ranging)	grain
Fish (including shell fish)	Beans (even if soaked overnight in lime, slow cooked)
Soy and Tofu (unprocessed)	
Dairy	

Try to eat only super low-fat, free-ranging, organically grown meat and poultry. If you can't afford free-ranging, then choose the lowest fat version available.

All you have to do is divide your plate up as follows: 35% protein (super lean meat, fish, poultry, or low-fat tofu), 35% complex carbs (veggies – not grains) and 30% fat (from nuts, seeds, avocados and healthy oils such as olive and canola) and fruits. Fruits are placed in a separate category because they must be eaten apart, as a meal unto themselves (the digestive enzymes needed to digest fruit are very different than those that digest other foods). Eating fruits with other foods will cause gas and bloating, and affect the assimilation of other foods. So, what do restaurants do? Of course, place fruits as a garnishment with every entrée. Save fruit for your snacks.

Top Ten Eating Tips

1) Eat a big breakfast, predominately made up of protein. (For every 100 calories of protein you eat, 20 calories are burned in the digestion process).

2) Eat good snacks. Don't wait until you are hungry; by then, you have low blood sugar and the brain is screaming for food – especially in the form of sugar. Eat high-protein and/or high fiber snacks, like nuts or seeds. According to Durk Pearson and Sandy Shaw, protein, eaten thirty to forty-five minutes before main meals, can further reduce appetite. (Amino acids in the protein are converted within this time to norepinephrine – the appetite-inhibiting neurotransmitter.)

3) Eat one or two vegetables with every meal. (Please don't count French fries).

4) Get your calcium from soymilk or dark green vegetables. Avoid regular milk.

5) Don't eat any potatoes except yams or sweet potatoes. White potatoes have a glycemic index higher than table sugar.

6) Eat a high quality protein with every meal.

7) When eating grains, eat only 100% whole grains. In moderation!

8) Eat fruit separately from other meals.

9) Drink six-8 ounces glasses of water per day (women), eight-8 ounce glasses per day (men), but not within 15 minutes before or after eating; otherwise, the saliva in your mouth is diluted and the digestion process is delayed.

10) Reduce or eliminate white sugar. Remember that fat-free usually means lots of sugar – a bad trade-off.

CHAPTER FIFTEEN – THE CAFFEINE DIET IN PRACTICE

Thank you for your coffee, seignor. I shall miss that when we leave Casablanca. - Ingrid Bergman

Caffeine: different doses for different tasks

It is important for you to learn how to use caffeine effectively so you can access all the benefits that is has to offer. One important aspect about caffeine is that the extent of its benefits is dependent on many variables. Caffeine may help you to listen to the radio and talk on the phone at the same time. Change the conditions slightly you won't have any more ability to concentrate studying if a noisy dog is barking outside your window.

The effects of caffeine are also dose dependent. It may only take you 50 mg. of caffeine to feel you mood lift, but it may take you 100 mg. to reduce your appetite, or 300 mg. to enhance your athletic performance. You can look at the table in Appendix "H" for typical caffeine values, and that should help you get a rough estimate of how much caffeine you will need for different tasks. It is important as always to remember though that results can be different from person to person.

Our Version of "a Cup"

I want to remind you again that throughout this book when I use the words a cup of coffee I am talking about 100 mg. of caffeine. Typically, this amount is equivalent one small cup of coffee, 1/3 cup of a large glass of coffee, or 3 cups of black tea, or 3 cans of caffeinated soda.

About Dosage

People respond to caffeine differently. We will look at how two people respond to different doses of caffeine. We know that genetic factors and the overall health of a person will affect the way they respond to caffeine. If person one is in ill health and person two is healthy and caffeine sensitivity, they respond to 200 mg. of caffeine differently. Will caffeine keep each person up later in the night if they drink too much caffeine during the day? How much is too much caffeine for each person? What about avoid using it altogether?

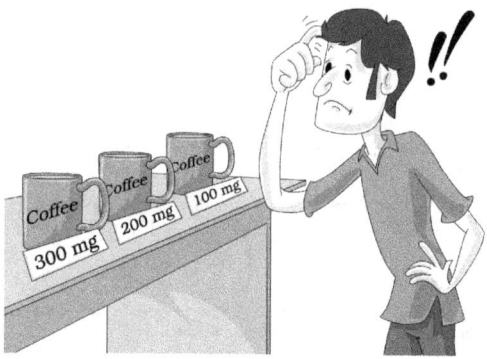

These are just some factors to take into consideration. We have already discussed the importance of experimenting to find out the correct dose for you. The best way to find answers is to use the self tests offered in this book. They give you an exact dose of caffeine at one time which makes it much easier to determine the results.

You can achieve similar results if you are consistent with the amount of caffeine you digest, and if you follow a schedule for the purpose of observation. Due to the complex nature of caffeine's effects, and the numbers of variables involved, we suggest you take the self tests. They will help you to get the most out of your caffeine use.

As we mentioned herein there is a very small percentage of the population that respond negatively to any amount of caffeine. These people become agitated, experience palpitations, or can't sleep well even when consuming minute amounts of caffeine.

Caffeine is safe for most healthy adults. We know this from the many long-term studies done on thousands of people that caffeine does not contribute to cardiovascular disease, cancer, or mortality . . . and may, in fact, provide significant benefits.

We still suggest that you be sure to consult your doctor before undertaking the programs described in this book. This is especially important if you are being treated for any medical condition.

How Much and When to Use Caffeine

In most people 100 mg. of caffeine is enough to produce sustained benefits in mood, cognition, and exercise endurance. We regard 100 mg. as the basic dose of caffeine. The basic dose is what you can safely take while experimenting with caffeine. You will understand better how it works to improve your mind and your mood as well as help you gain control of your appetite once you've spent some time experimenting.

It is not important to worry about why you may require more or less caffeine than someone else. You will find the amount that works best for you. It is important for you to know that if you follow the instructions laid out in this book, this program will unquestionably work for you.

Timing is The Key to the Caffeine Diet

One major impact on how successful you will be on this diet is timing.

Your first dose in the morning is to take caffeine right after breakfast. There are several reasons for this. Breakfast should be your biggest meal of the day. Taking caffeine before this big meal suppresses the appetite and will result in eating almost double the amount of calories during the rest of the day. Breakfast should be protein based. Protein triggers the release of norepinephrine which boosts mood and energy. Carbohydrates trigger the release of serotonin, which is the calming agent. Also, carbs trigger an insulin reaction approximately 20 minutes after eating, resulting in sugar / sweets craving, and binge eating.

You can combat the craving by taking caffeine immediately after your breakfast. The result will be that caffeine's appetite-suppressant properties will reach 75% of its peak properties at approximately the same time you would usually experience the insulin reaction, or sugar cravings. This will help you to regain control of your appetite and be ready to begin the day. This success first thing in the morning sets the tone for the whole day.

Your second dose is used to combat the mid-morning sugar cravings. You will need to experiment to find out what time this occurs for you. In most people it happens halfway between breakfast and lunch (normally 10:30 a.m. to 11:00 a.m.). You want to take your second dose of caffeine 15-20 minutes before this time.

Your third dose should be right after lunch. This dose is for the same reasons as the first dose: to fight off the cravings created by consumption of carbohydrates. We suggest a good size lunch. (the focus of lunch should be salad with some protein – tofu, chicken, etc.). Protein also triggers the brain to shut down the appetite center. This dose will enable you to work focused and fast right through the post-lunch let down most people experience.

Your fourth dose will be 15-20 minutes before your mid-afternoon sugar craving. For most people this will be 2:30 p.m. to 3:00 p.m. Caffeine will suppress your appetite, which is a desired affect at this time of day. It will also give you more energy, sharpen thinking, and help memory retention. This dose will also help carry you through the rest of the day at your maximum efficiency.

Your fifth dose will be 15-20 minutes before dinner. We suggest that dinner be the smallest of your meals. This fifth dose will work to control the number of calories you consume. Many people eat out for most of their meals. We don't recommend this as there are many preservatives and flavorings added to food which trigger appetite and affect the hypothalamus (slowing metabolism). Many times a person will consume the majority of their calories at dinner. This does not allow the body enough time to burn off the calories before sleep. Also, if dinner includes carbohydrates, the body will not process glucose correctly when you sleep. The fifth dose is your last dose of the day. It is important as a defense against the temptations of bingeing. For most people half way between dinner and bed time they experience another craving.

Your sixth preventative action You can't use caffeine any later to fight off food cravings because it is too close to bedtime. The recommendation here is to take a careful, close look at our list of 27 approved snacks. These protein-based snacks, which are about 100 calories each, will not only provide healthy calories, but protein triggers the release of CCK which signals the hypothalamus to shut down the appetite center. The list of snacks can be found in Appendix "C." It is a good idea to have these snacks readily available so you have the ammunition to win the fight against cravings and bingeing. Whatever is most available is what you'll eat when you're hungry or craving sugar or sweets. If your shelves and refrigerator are stocked with ice cream and cookies, then you'll choose those. If it's on our approved list, then you'll make a much wiser, healthier choice. It is important that you remember to take your snack before (15-30 minutes) the hunger pangs/cravings occur. For most people, this occurs at 8:00 – 8:00 p.m.

Caffeine: Not a Treat

For our purposes we are using caffeine as a medicine. It you add milk (cows) to coffee for example it will lose its fat burning and metabolism boosting properties. However, now there is an option when it comes to sugar. Naturolose (see appendix) is a healthy alternative, and is the only sugar that can be used if you desire to attain all the positive effects of caffeine.

Where to Start

We suggest starting with 100 mgs. of caffeine five times per day. You will need to experiment as you are already aware. You will know how caffeine affects your appetite, focus, energy and mood from your experimentation. We recommend using a coffee that has a label that clearly tell how much caffeine you are getting from a teaspoon, or ounce, or measured cup. You need to know exactly how much caffeine you are starting with and how much you are adding to you beginning dosage. Labels should also provide you with the specific brewing process and bean type which affect the caffeine dose.

When doing your experiments, note that even very small doses of 25 mg. to 50 mg. a day can confer considerable benefits on sensitive people, or those who have little experience with caffeine. For most people, using more caffeine will be perfectly safe.

Studies done on military personnel have shown that a person can take 600 mg. of caffeine to help them maintain speed of reactions and visual and auditory vigilance. The dose also proved to be effective in sustaining physical endurance. This is the one time during the day when it is okay to take more than your normal dosage. (From 300-600 mg. of caffeine 15-30 minutes before exercising). The military studies concluded that caffeine is safe. They went on to say that caffeine was their choice for helping to counteract cognitive deficits.

Studies have found the following:

1) Low doses have long term positive effects on mood.
2) Low doses improve memory.
3) Low doses improve reaction time.
4) Low doses increase attention span.
5) Low to moderate doses minimize the risk of adverse side effects
6) Low to moderate doses minimize the risk over-caffeineating.
7) Moderate doses enable maximum physical exertion.
8) Moderate doses help to fight the effects of fatigue and sleep deprivation.

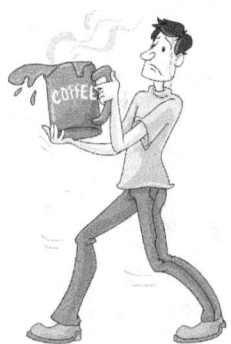

The Diverse Benefits of Caffeine

When you're fatigued or bored, caffeine restores your energy and attention to normal levels. If you are already alert, caffeine augments your abilities and helps you to perform at higher levels.

Recently, researchers have begun to compare these two effects in individual studies. In one such study, researchers determined that caffeine delivered many benefits in both situations. It showed that when people were impaired by fatigue or lack of sleep the benefits were felt more significantly. The effects on shortening reaction time were the same whether the person was fatigued or well rested. It seemed the most important variable in the power of caffeine was its ability to help the subject whether they were well rested or not.

Caffeine is known to be beneficial in many ways. In the morning caffeine can improve one's mood and focus, while later in the day reducing cravings by keeping blood sugar levels balanced. Caffeine can improve short-term memory and acts as an appetite suppressant. When exercising, caffeine increases endurance and also lowers blood pressure by increasing sodium excretion.

How Much is that Cup in the Window

One reason caffeine pills or capsules can be a good idea is you know exactly how much caffeine you are getting. You are eliminating the guess work of determining how much caffeine is in a cup of coffee.

There are other options as well; including but not limited to; caffeinated mints, caffeinated chewing gums, caffeinated vanilla ice cream, and caffeinated waters. One problem with these other options is that they typically fail to reveal how much caffeine they contain. Caffeine is a drug and you want to know how much you are taking.

The primary source of caffeine in America is Arabica beans. This accounts for 75% of all caffeine consumption worldwide. It is used exclusively in making gourmet coffees. Different varieties of arabica contain slightly different amounts of caffeine averaging about 1.1 percent caffeine by weight. Coffea robusta accounts for the remaining 25% of worldwide consumption. Coffea robusta has twice the caffeine content by weight averages about 2.2 percent. Coffea robusta is used only in the cheapest blends.

For our purposes we will assume that the coffee you will be drinking is made from arabica beans. However it is important to note that if you have coffee made from robusta beans, it will have twice the caffeine content of the same sized portion of coffee from Arabica beans.

The Problem With Using Cola

Your body will react to neutralize acidic drinks such as colas with alkaline blood buffers. When this process occurs other acidic waste products continually produced by the body are not being neutralized. This includes acetic acid, lactic acid (a byproduct of exercise – the side stitch), carbonic acid, uric acid, and fatty acids. When the body's supply of alkaline buffers is defeated, these toxic acidic waste products accumulate in the body causing significant health damage.

The body uses calcium to convert the poisonous liquid phosphoric acid in colas into more stable solid phosphates. This process leads to the development of urinary infections and kidney stones. This occurs because the phosphates may form into calcium deposits, but the real culprit may be the high level of phosphoric acid. This is a primary ingredient in colas.

As our bodies become increasingly acidic our cells must adapt. They do this through an internal evolutionary process and become more like plant cells, which have a high tendency to become cancer cells. Routine consumption of soft drinks can also result in bone loss.

This does not even begin to address the issue of sugars, calories, and additives.

Caffeinated Chewing Gum

As we discussed, there are many new non-traditional sources of caffeine. These caffeinated products are growing more and more popular. One of the more promising products is caffeinated chewing gum. Stay Alert, a brand of caffeinated gum contains 50 mg. of caffeine per stick. Studies have shown the gum effectively restores alertness and dramatically increases performance levels. Eighty percent of the caffeine in the gum is absorbed in 5 minutes. This results in a faster mental and physical boost than the same dose of caffeine consumed in a cup of coffee. The gums other advantages are fairly obvious: It's easily portable requiring no fluids. It also delivers caffeine in finely graduated-doses.

Caffeine Pills

Caffeine pills have a stronger effect per milligram of caffeine, which means we use less caffeine when taking pills than when drinking coffee. Decreasing the dose of caffeine eliminates any unusual adverse side effects that some people experience.

It is also true that coffee can upset your stomach by increasing acid production (less true with organic coffees). Pure caffeine delivers the most punch with the lowest chance of any adverse consequences.

People tend to use pills when they are already feeling fatigued. Many students and truck drivers who are pulling all-nighters use caffeine pills. Few people try them under normal circumstances; therefore few people have the experience of seeing what the pills can do when they are well rested. People also tend to use caffeine pills for emergency situations, and they never get to experience the sustained advantages that pills can provide.

Decaf

Some research suggests that a portion of caffeine's benefits are lost to chlorogenic acid found in coffee. Decaffeination removes much of the chlorogenic acid. If you still want to enjoy the experience of drinking coffee but also get the biggest boost in performance from caffeine try using caffeine pills and drinking decaf.

More on Tolerance and Caffeine

Research shows that tolerance doesn't negate many of caffeine's effects. However it is clear that caffeine causes a physical dependence to occur. When we use any substance that promotes physical and cerebral abilities, and then suddenly discontinue its use, we can expect to experience withdrawal symptoms.

The withdrawal symptoms of caffeine have been well recognized for over a century. Headaches are the most common symptom associated with quitting caffeine too quickly. Other symptoms can include sleepiness, irritability, or even flu like symptoms such as muscle aches and nausea. These symptoms can be reduced by gradually cutting down on caffeine over a week or more.

The more caffeine you are taking the stronger will be your physical dependence. The stronger your physical dependence the worse your withdrawal symptoms will be if you suddenly stop using caffeine. Even if you are drinking as little as one cup of coffee a day, you might feel slightly uncomfortable if you quit drinking coffee abruptly. Approximately thirty percent of people who suddenly stop caffeine use will experience withdrawal symptoms.

Caffeinism

Some researchers say that because people enjoy the effects of caffeine, it can create a psychological dependence. When this psychological dependence combines with a physical dependence to interfere with a person's life, the resulting syndrome is called "caffeinism," a recognized psychiatric condition.

Sufferers of caffeinism continue to use excessive amounts of caffeine even though it is adversely affecting them. A person who takes excessive doses of caffeine in an effort to intensify the mood and physical benefits of the drug might also be diagnosed with caffeinism. This syndrome is uncommon but if you suspect it you should markedly reduce or even eliminate caffeine intake and seek professional counseling if necessary.

Symptoms of Caffeine Withdrawal

1) Headaches
2) Irritability
3) Anxiety
4) Bad moods
5) Difficulty working
6) Depression
7) Difficulty concentrating
8) Fatigue Sleepiness, drowsiness
9) Flu-like symptoms

The Placebo Theory

One theory is that caffeine's benefits are a creation of our mind. The researchers in this study argued that because a period of abstinence from caffeine initiates withdrawal symptoms the supposed "improvements" in performance and are simply the result of feeding our caffeine habit. They say what we are really feeling is the feeling of getting back to normal. However study after study has disproven this theory.

All the benefits of caffeine are experienced in people who aren't regular caffeine users and therefore obviously are not experiencing withdrawal symptoms when they stop using it. The benefits are also found in people who regularly use caffeine but have not been deprived of it prior to the testing period.

Caffeine abstinence can make you tired or depressed but it does not cause any detrimental effects on athletic, mental, or psychomotor performance. There are no "withdrawal-related deficits" to reduce.

Caffeine and Fatigue

Caffeine has the power to help us take charge of our biological clocks. Taking charge of our biological clocks enables us to feel refreshed and well rested in conditions where we would otherwise feel exhausted. Caffeine increases muscular endurance and decreases fatigue. This ability allows for an increase in the time during which we can do physical work before becoming exhausted. There are three ways in which caffeine effectively "makes time" by:

1) extending the period during which people can perform work.
2) Caffeine sharpens specific abilities including alertness, reasoning, verbal fluency, memory, reaction time, and attention span. It also mitigates depression mental confusion.
3) Caffeine increases muscular endurance and decreases fatigue.

Caffeine and the Fight Against Fatigue

Early in the 20th century experiments on caffeine and how it affected human performance were conducted. These early experiments concluded that caffeine facilitates performance in fatigued people. They also showed that daily doses of less than 700 mg. will not disturb sleep for most people.

Caffeine works to fight against fatigue in many ways. Caffeine reverses the depression and boredom which often accompany fatigue, or prolonged sleep deprivation. This practice of using caffeine to fend off exhaustion has been in use for many decades. During World War II many veterans recount how coffee played an important role in helping them remain alert during the long hours of wakefulness required in military life.

In modern warfare the action on the field of battle goes on 24 hours a day thanks the introduction of new technology. In order for military personnel to meet these demands they use coffee. Studies have been done on the role of caffeine and how it affects performance caused by sleep disruption. This is especially important in people who must perform heavy physical demands. The studies concluded that caffeine is the best agent available to counteract fatigue in battlefield conditions. They also concluded that caffeine was beneficial for civilian life as well. Many other occupations require long hours of wakefulness, and caffeine can be used for people in those professions as well and for anyone who is sleep deprived.

One study done on subjects who had been without sleep for 48 hours, used doses of 150 mg. 300 mg., or 600 mg. of caffeine. There were improvements observed at all dosage levels. The 600 mg. dose improved cognitive performance, alertness, and self-assessments of mood as much as a 20 mg. dose of amphetamine did, caffeine obviously having fewer side effects than amphetamines. The study showed that caffeine may help postpone sleep up to 12 hours.

Metabolism and Sleep Deprivation

When you're tired or sleep deprived your metabolic rate drops. Studies show caffeine increases the metabolic rates of sleep-deprived subjects to normal levels. This helps a person to overcome lethargy and restores them to levels of a well-rested person. Another study was conducted on people who didn't sleep for two days. These subjects were given varying doses of caffeine. Researchers looked closely at how caffeine affects mood, alertness, and mental clarity. The study found that relatively high doses of caffeine reversed the effects of sleep deprivation on both alertness and mood.

In sleep-deprived people, caffeine reversed conditions in several tests of vigor, fatigue, and confusion. Peak effects began to wane after about 4 hours, however the higher dose of caffeine produced significant, long-lasting, beneficial mood enhancement in the sleep deprived persons. These effects were noted even after 48 hours.

More recent studies proved that higher doses of caffeine actually reverse the effects of prolonged sleep deprivation. Another observation was that even the large 600 mg. dose did not increase levels of heart palpitation, headaches, perspiration, or upset stomach in subjects.

Curing the Post Lunch Slump

Most people experience a slump after eating lunch that makes them long for an afternoon nap. Many people fail to realize that it's not just in their imagination, or the result of a boring job. This syndrome has been documented by scientists for years.

Recent studies have shown that certain slumps in performance after eating a meal can be found independent of time of day. Many studies have shown scores on tasks requiring thinking and attention declined after subjects had eaten lunch, while there was no change in the performance of subjects who hadn't eaten.

We know that eating causes many changes in the body. Digestion takes a great deal of bodily resources. Scientists have speculated that an increase in blood glucose or a release of gastrointestinal hormones such as insulin or serotonin may be responsible.

The good news found by scientific studies has proven caffeine can combat the afternoon slump. Studies have found, in fact, that if caffeine is used correctly it can eliminate the effects of the afternoon slump entirely.

Many people experience a tendency for their mind to wander after eating a midday meal. The tasks requiring sustained attention suffer the greatest decline in performance after lunch.

One study, hoping to find out if caffeine can combat this problem, evaluated university students. The students were given caffeine tablets equivalent to 3 mg. per kilogram of body weight, then asked to perform vigilance tests with and without caffeine.

Caffeine improved performance before and after lunch, showing far greater improvement after lunch. Breakfast and lunch produce different patterns of effects on performance. Caffeine appears to interact differently with the declines in performance after each meal.

Even though caffeine can completely eliminate the slump most people experience after eating lunch, it has a lesser effect after eating breakfast. Breakfast doesn't affect alertness or attention span but it appears to affect logical reasoning when it is carbohydrate-based.

Caffeine delivers relief from the bad mood many people experience along with the post lunch slump. People who take caffeine after lunch feel significantly more content, happier, and more interested in their work. Studies also show when people eat a substantial meal they feel calmer if they have caffeine with the meal. There was an increase in tension observed in subjects took caffeine but skipped breakfast.

Evening meals produce a barely noticeable slump when it was not a big (no more than 600 mg.) or heavy on carbs (more than 35%). Under these circumstances, the evening meal also creates fewer changes in cognitive performance, mood, and behavior. This is good news because you can't really caffeinate after dinner without effecting sleep patterns.

Caffeine and Shift Work

Night workers often experience fatigue and lack of concentration during their shift. Anyone whose job requires them to do shift work can tell you about the symptoms they experience. When a person changes from a morning shift to a night shift it creates much stress on the body. In many ways, arriving for work on a new shift is like getting off a plane in another country. You are being forced to work at the lowest point of your energies.

It is common for shift workers to be inattentive, forgetful, and slow to respond. Another reason for this is that when a person sleeps during the day rather than at night they get on average 2 hours less of sleep.

The real problem occurs because just about the time the body has acclimated to the changes caused by working a night shift, most people have to change back to a day or evening shift. This keeps shift workers in a perpetual state of "jet lag".

Caffeine can combat the symptoms of fatigue and lack of sleep. Caffeine, when used properly, can bring shift workers up to speed at their jobs. It makes them as alert and quick to respond as they are during the day. Caffeine can also help to alleviate the crankiness often experienced by shift workers.

One of the earliest studies of caffeine's usefulness in sustaining wakefulness and reducing sleepiness showed profound results. This study proved that the benefits of 200 to 400 mg. of caffeine were equal to or greater than a 3-hour nap taken between midnight and 3 A.M.

One study looked to find out if caffeine's effects on alertness and sleepiness were different for people who used a small or moderate amount of caffeine, as compared with those who use a great deal. Subjects were split into two groups: those who regularly consumed two or fewer caffeinated drinks a day and those who regularly consumed five to seven caffeinated drinks a day. The study showed that doses of 200 mg. to 400 mg. of caffeine significantly reduced physiological sleepiness. They also found it improved the ability to sustain wakefulness at times of marked sleepiness. Identical doses of caffeine had a similar effect on both light and heavy caffeine users. The effects lasted several hours, which is important for workers who sometimes must sustain performance throughout the night and keep going the next day on little or no sleep. The study showed that alertness was heightened to a level of those on a regular day shift. A moderate dose (300 mg.) produced benefits for 5+ hours. A high dose (600 mg.) provided 7+ hours of benefit.

Caffeine and Driving Alertness

Taking the right dose of caffeine will enable the tired driver to experience an increase in reaction time and the ability to make quick decisions will improve. It has been estimated that there are 100,000 highway accidence per year due to tired drivers, and over 3,000 deaths. Feeling more clear-headed, calm, and alert while driving is very important for obvious reasons.

Thank You and Good Night

Caffeine's most universally recognized benefit is its ability to keep you awake when you want to stay awake. We know that caffeine can also keep you awake when you want to be asleep. Scientific studies have proven that caffeine can create problems with sleep. One study of over 200 subjects noted that almost 50% of those surveyed said that a strong cup of coffee before bedtime would most definitely interfere with falling asleep.

A second study found that when night shift workers consumed 200 mg. of caffeine after midnight they remained awake through the night. The study showed taking another 200 mg. at 7 A.M. helped them to restore alertness through the following day.

A third study found that 42% of the house staff at one hospital admitted to killing at least one patient by making a fatigue-related mistake. The use of caffeine in these circumstances could literally save lives.

The following factors determine the effect caffeine will have on falling and staying asleep:

1. The milligrams of caffeine.
2. The number of hours before bedtime.
3. The rate at which a person metabolizes caffeine.
4. General sensitivity to caffeine
5. Specific individual sensitivity to caffeine
6. The regular amount consumed daily.

Generally speaking, people who limit their intake of caffeine believe it would keep them from falling asleep at night if consumed too close to bed time. One study showed two-thirds of women who drank only one or two cups of coffee a day found that a cup consumed shortly before bedtime interfered with their sleep. This same study showed that only one fourth of subjects who drank twice that amount daily reported any interference with sleep if they consumed coffee prior to bedtime.

This study raised many questions about people who do not experience insomnia from drinking coffee and those who do. It made scientists wonder if people who are heavy coffee drinkers build up a tolerance to caffeine's effects on sleep. It is a difficult question to answer

Caffeine and Sleep

Caffeine has a wide range of effects on the ability of a person to fall asleep. There are a small number of people who actually use caffeine to fall asleep. These people seem to respond to caffeine in a different manner than most of the population. Another small percentage of people actually sleep too much when they use caffeine. This is a condition known as hypersomnia. It is important to keep these findings in mind when you are being advised whether you should or should not be using caffeine bedtime.

There is no question that for the average person caffeine taken before bedtime generally delays the onset of sleep. It is up to the individual to determine what "before bedtime" means, as each person reacts differently to caffeine. One person can safely take caffeine up to three hours before bed where another needs to stop using caffeine six hours before bed.

To find out more specifically how caffeine affects you we suggest that you record not only the quantity of your sleep but the quality. Use a scale of your choosing to measure the quality of sleep you get each night. For some people caffeine might not interfere with the time that they fall asleep, but it will cause them to be restless and not get a good night's rest.

Caffeine and Aging

Caffeine affects middle-aged and older people differently than it does younger people. Older individuals experience more powerful benefits. As people age they tend to sleep less and less. Between the ages of twenty-five and seventy-five most people lose two hours of sleep per night.

As we age it becomes very important not to do anything that will interfere with the amount of sleep we are getting.

For our purposes, we suggest to stop all caffeine intake (soda, coffee, pills, and some medications that contain caffeine) after dinner or approximately 7:00 P.M. If you still experience any difficulty in falling asleep then try stopping your caffeine consumption at 4:00 P.M.

Even if you are highly sensitive to caffeine you can likely find a way to enjoy caffeine's benefits and avoid the unwanted side effects. We suggest you change the source from which you are getting your caffeine. Try using black or even green tea. A cup of black tea the same size of a cup of coffee has only about 40 to 50 mg. and a cup of green tea has only about 10 to 15 mg.

Caffeinated soft drinks are another relatively low-dose source of caffeine. People who are sensitive to caffeine's effects may become more alert and energetic after drinking a single, small caffeinated soda without disturbing their sleep at night.

Finding Your Cut Off Point

A 6 ounce cup of filter drip coffee contains nearly 150 mg. of caffeine. A large mug of filter drip coffee can deliver 400 mg. or more. If you experience problems that you associate with caffeine - for example, insomnia, jitteriness, or rapid heartbeat - then you might consider how much caffeine you are actually consuming. You may be consuming 300-600 mg. of caffeine when you think it is only 100-150 mg. Keep changing the amount of your dose until you pinpoint your personal caffeine cutoff point. You will then know exactly how much caffeine you can take without experiencing negative side effects.

Kicking the Habit

It is easy for a physician to tell his or her patient to stop taking caffeine. Many people experience difficulty when it comes to really trying to cut caffeine out of their daily routine. Part of the difficulty lies in the fact that many substances like tea and chocolate also contain caffeine and are therefore off limits.

It takes approximately a week for all the caffeine to be out of your system. Once you are rid of all caffeine you lose all tolerance to caffeine's effects. After seven days you will no longer be experiencing any withdrawal symptoms

In order to minimize the unpleasant withdrawal symptoms we recommend stepping down your dose. We suggest that you add the number 2 to however many cups of coffee you consume each day. If you drink 5 cups of coffee a day expect that the tapering down process will take 7 days. Each day attempt to decrease your caffeine intake by one cup and the final two days you will be caffeine free.

You can expect to experience some withdrawal symptoms. The severity of the withdrawal experience is unique to each person. Generally it is dependent on how physically dependent you are on caffeine and your unique genetic makeup.

Obviously the person who consumes an average of 600 mg. of caffeine per day is going to have a harder time quitting than the person who only consumes 100 mg. per day.

When it comes to your genetic makeup, certain people are more likely to develop a physical dependence. They tend to experience more intense withdrawal symptoms when trying to stop. You will learn for yourself the degree of withdrawal that you experience when you first try to detoxify from caffeine.

Most people don't experience much trouble when attempting to cut down caffeine use from higher daily doses like 600 mg. to a daily dose of 100 mg. The hardest part for most people comes when the approach the final step from 100 mg. of caffeine a day to none at all.

If you are one of the few people who experience significant discomfort when doing this, you can combat the experience by taking a very small dose of caffeine about 15 mg. when you feel the discomfort. This small dose won't greatly interfere with your step-down program, and it may make you feel a great deal better.

The Hidden Caffeine

There are many sources of caffeine that people are unaware of. For example, many over the counter headache remedies contain caffeine. When attempting to follow a caffeine withdrawal program, be sure you are aware of any of these hidden sources. Many carbonated soft drinks also contain caffeine. Try to avoid using them as they will sabotage your stepping-down program. It really does take discipline and determination to do any type of detoxification process.

A Closer Look at Caffeine and Jet Lag

Jet lag affects everyone differently. There are a few common symptoms that most people experience. These include; fatigue, sleep disturbances, insomnia, mild depression, irritability, gastrointestinal distress, and headaches. Other, less common, symptoms include dehydration, disorientation, anxiety, impaired coordination, slower reaction time, and poor concentration.

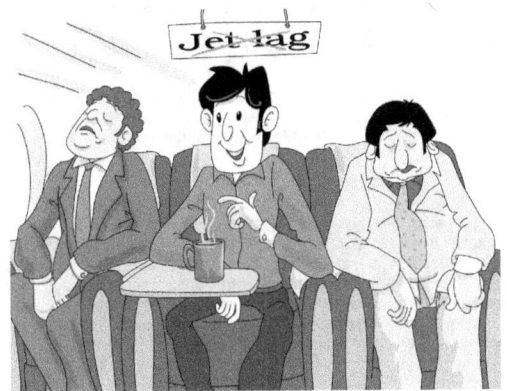

Studies have proven that jet lag seriously impairs a subject's ability to perform mental and physical tasks. Caffeine counteracts the most damaging symptoms of jet lag, such as: Reduction in dynamic strength, disorientation, reduction in muscle power and capacity, Loss of appetite, stomach distress, prolonged reaction time, decreased short-term memory, decreased concentration, Insomnia, higher injury rates, fatigue.

After You Land

The most important part of fighting jet lag takes place after you land. This means staying awake the entire first day and going to bed around 10 P.M. or 11 P.M. local time. In order to accomplish this you must use caffeine to keep your body awake and your mind alert. It will take a few days in the new time zone to become acclimated. Caffeine will also be signaling your body to reset your clock to local time.

If you have followed the schedule of caffeine withdrawal prior to your travels you will have had two entire days where you have been free of caffeine before you leave on your trip. This is enough time to dramatically increase your sensitivity to caffeine's effects. So taking a cup of coffee or a Thermo Power Boost® tablet on arrival will start to signal your hypothalamus to begin resetting your body's clock.

These tablets come in very precise 100 mg. dosage. And you will be able to take your dose even if the stewardesses are no longer serving close to landing. Take the pills or coffee 15 minutes before landing. This first dose should get you through baggage and the process of getting to your hotel.

Once you are comfortably situated, have a meal that includes both protein and carbohydrates. After your meal it is time for another dose of caffeine.

We recommend that in order to reset your clock you get out into the sunshine and get some exercise; perhaps a walk around whatever city you are visiting. Remember, even if you are feeling tired, don't take a nap.

Every three to four hours continue taking whatever dose of caffeine you have determined works for you. Remember to stop taking any caffeine source once you reach your nightly cut off point. If you follow all the advice given you should be able to fall asleep at around 10 P.M. or 11 P.M.

We highly suggest that you take advantage of caffeine's ability to help you overcome jet lag. You must follow a program such as the one we have outline in this chapter to be successful. By planning ahead you can minimize any discomforts of caffeine withdrawal.

When to Travel

Studies have shown it is better to immediately switch your routine to a new time schedule when traveling. This is exactly what our caffeine-based jet lag program helps you to do. This really aids in decreasing the effects of jet lag. For example, when athletes travel to other countries they often arrive in the morning. They are advised by their trainers to stay up through the day and go to bed that night at local time. Athletes also exercise in order to help cut down the length of time that jet lag causes impairments. One study found that exercising outdoors helped the resynchronization process more than those who stayed indoors and did not exercise.

CHAPTER SIXTEEN - CAFFEINE, CREATIVITY, AND MENTAL PERFORMANCE

As soon as coffee is in your stomach, there is a general commotion. Ideas begin to move, similes arise, the paper is covered. Coffee is your ally and writing ceases to be a struggle - Honoré de Balzac

Here, we will be further exploring how caffeine, when taken by a well-rested person, can enhance reasoning ability, reaction time, memory, alertness and attention span.

Decades of research have shown that caffeine actually makes you smarter. Most people who use caffeine regularly find that they are sharper and quicker on an on-going basis. They also have found that the degree of improvement is directly proportional to the amount of caffeine used.

Caffeine's power to increase intelligence does not wear off over time and doesn't require us to take larger doses of the drug. Research shows that low to moderate amounts of caffeine produce an almost instant improvement in intelligence tests. The same dose will results in the providing the same improvement indefinitely.

Caffeine and Mental Performance

Studies have shown that we are more or less stimulated by caffeine depending on our state of mind and body prior to use. The following is a list of factors that influence arousal:

Loud noises
Overall Health
Fatigue
Illness
Personality type (extrovert/introvert)
Amount of caffeine consumed

When it comes to understanding the relationship between the level of arousal and the level of performance. The following guidelines apply:

1. Small doses of caffeine confer some benefits.
2. Medium to large doses of caffeine confers more pronounced benefits.
3. Very large doses of caffeine do not increase benefits further and may even cause decrements.

There are other variables to consider as well. For one person a "small" dose might be what another person considers a "medium" dose. In what we will call low-arousal people there is a tendency to be more outgoing and impulsive. This group of people tends to look towards outside stimulus for excitement. High-arousal people are generally introverts and tend to be less impulsive and not seek out high levels of external stimulation. One study shows that this group is more resistant to the effects of caffeine and other drugs.

If your arousal level is already high, you probably won't get any benefits from larger doses of caffeine. In this state you may actually lose the benefits conferred by lower doses.

Contradicting Evidence

In doing our research we have come across countless studies that support the case that caffeine decreases mental performance. There is an equal amount of research showing that caffeine increases mental performance.

Studies found improvements in mental function in people who were in a low to moderate state of arousal. They also showed that there were no improvements and even some decrements when arousal levels become too high. Another scientist also found that people with a lower tendency to be impulsive got more from caffeine than did those who were highly impulsive.

Arousal Factors and Performance: Customizing Your Dose

Arousal theory provides a look at how caffeine affects the mind. There are many complex factors that contribute to the contradictory findings:

Dose: Large amounts of caffeine can result in a person going past the optimum arousal levels. When this happens the benefits of caffeine are diminished. Many of the early studies failed to understand this relationship between dose and arousal. Researchers were confused by when studies showed lower doses of caffeine improved performance and higher doses impaired performance. The same results were found on attention, problem-solving, and memory task.

Baseline Arousal: Baseline arousal is a person's state of excitation or stimulation prior to beginning the performance of a task. If a person is already aroused they can become over stimulated when asked to perform highly arousing tasks. This over stimulation generates errors in tests of mental abilities.

Relative Task Complexity: The more complex a task is the more arousal levels are increased. This can contribute to over-stimulation and impair performance. Each person will, however, have a different idea of what constitutes a complex task. A task that appears relatively complex for one person may be simple for the next person.

Some people can take on these tasks quicker when taking caffeine. When impulsive people use caffeine they have shown significant improvements on IQ tests and other tests on memory and psychomotor performance. People who are not impulsive show little or no benefit in these areas when they use caffeine. These results support the findings of the arousal theory. Take these findings into consideration for your own situations. If you tend to be more withdrawn and have more of an introvert personality you should consider taking less caffeine. In your case less may well be more.

A Complex Issue

We still don't fully understand all the way in which caffeine affects the adenosine neurotransmitter system. We can clearly see that it affects dopamine levels, catecholamine, and adrenaline systems, but it is a complex issue that needs more research.

It is a difficult task for researchers to determine if the benefits caffeine has on mental processes arise at the stage at which perceptual information enters the brain, or during the processing of this information. Also, whether it is during the decision as what action to take, or in the course of executing this decision. It seems more probably that the process occurs in all of these stages.

Your brain on caffeine

General Intelligence (GI) tests, like IQ tests are designed to estimate performance on specific tasks. People who do well on anyone of these tests tend to do well on all of them. The people who do well on the tests also tend to be people who achieve the most academically and in their jobs. Caffeine has been shown to improve performance on tests that measure rapid information processing, abstract reasoning, verbal fluency, computational ability, and memory. Based on this information one can safely say that caffeine raises IQ.

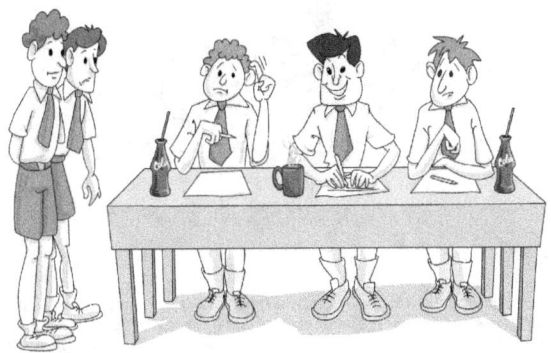

Caffeine also improves the ability to sustain attention over a long time, and enhances the ability to pay attention to two things at once. People make fewer mistakes and are able to accomplish more under the influence of caffeine. Studies have shown that caffeine also improves psychomotor performance.

In a test on the effects of low doses of caffeine, cognition studies showed that caffeine had a profound impact on verbal problem solving. Subjects who consumed doses of 75-150 mg. of caffeine scored correct answers at a considerably higher rate than those who didn't consume any caffeine prior to testing.

Another study found that caffeine improved performance on a semantic processing test as well as in calculation speed and error ratios. There was a dramatic improvement demonstrated in subject's performance on mental arithmetic.

We know that caffeine sharpens mental performance in all age groups; however in older people it improves performance on reasoning, memory, and reaction time more than it does the in younger people.

Caffeine and the Creative Mind

Caffeine is thought to affect the cerebrum which houses the thalamus, the part of the brain responsible for allowing sensory information to initiate physical response. The thalamus relays the sensory impulses of sight, hearing, touch, and taste to the cerebral cortex.

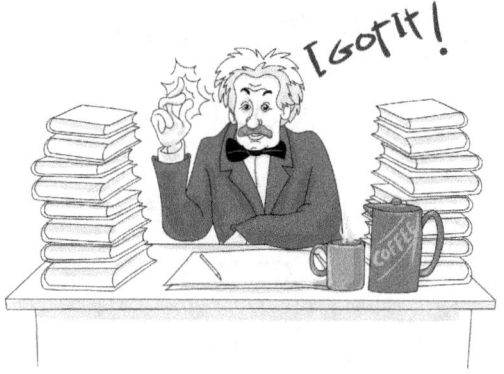

Studies have shown a relationship between caffeine and an improvement with the signal-to-noise ratio in what we see and hear. This improvement is responsible for creating a situation where, when listening or watching a video- or audiotape, the picture or sound jumps appears to stand out more vividly. Caffeine allows us zoom in on an object of interest and not be distracted by other stimuli present. We are able to pay attention better with the use of caffeine according to many studies done on the subject.

Caffeine and Vision

Caffeine improves vision. Tests have shown that after taking caffeine subjects see a greater numbers of faint twinkling stars as well as finer gradations in colors. The reason for this reaction is that caffeine decreases the intensity level of illumination, which the eye needs to recognize and discriminate between two matters.

Caffeine has also been proven to significantly lower the luminance threshold, which is the smallest amount of light a person can detect. Studies done on this subject showed a single cup coffee dramatically improved the ability to see details of objects in dim light. Caffeine also enabled subjects to notice more details in ordinary light.

Caffeine and the Artist

Caffeine improves visuo-spatial reasoning. For a painter, this means that it can help them create more complex compositions. If caffeine is used regularly, color discrimination increases significantly.

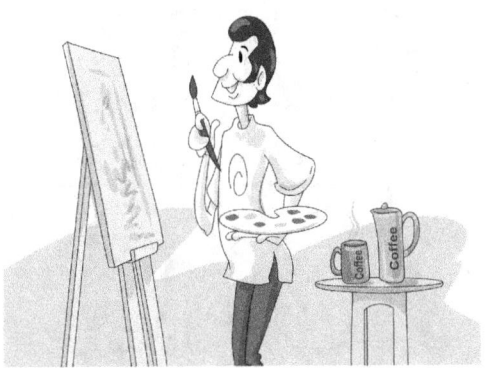

Studies done on this subject showed that when a person drank even one caffeinated drink a day they made nearly 60 percent fewer errors in distinguishing colors than people who rarely or never use caffeine. Other studies have shown that even the taste and smell of caffeine can have an effect on the senses. Smell and taste are both windows on the world and each has its own significant role for the artistic person.

Caffeine's ability to intensify flavor seems to have no impact on the central nervous system. Studies showed that when caffeine was given in pill form it failed to demonstrate any effect on taste. When a person is drinking coffee or tea, they are exposing the tongue to caffeine and altering the function of the taste buds. This is important because it will enable one to sense flavors more intensely.

Reaction Time

People who process information faster tend to have higher IQ's than people who process it slowly. We already know that caffeine increases virtually every measure of reaction time. Caffeine improves performance dramatically on tests of both simple and choice reaction time.

Driving an automobile requires good reaction in real time. This is another area where caffeine will improve your ability to make these important decisions. Having a quicker reaction time also enables a person who enjoys video games to be more successful. Studies have shown that even when regular caffeine users didn't consume any caffeine prior to testing they scored higher than non users on video games. This research leads one to believe that regular caffeine consumption has long-term benefits on the ability to make quick responses.

Caffeine vs. the Common Cold

In a recent experiment, college students were tested on memory and processingspeed at two different times. Once while healthy with no caffeine, the next time when they had colds and were retested after being given coffee, The researchers found no difference between those with colds and coffee and those who were healthy with no coffee. The experimenters only used the equivalent of one small cup of coffee (100 mg.).

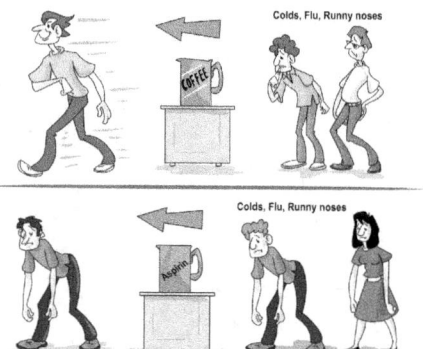

Vigilance

Caffeine has the ability to increase arousal levels and moderate doses of caffeine reduce boredom. Long-duration vigilance tests are particularly sensitive to the use of caffeine. When high doses of caffeine are used, initially performance on vigilance tasks is impaired. However as blood levels of caffeine decline, impairment reverses itself. Studies found that at this point the lower levels of caffeine remaining in the body actually improve performance.

Another study found that a subject's performance improved without loud noise but declined when noise was added. Caffeine didn't appear to improve performance when loud noise was a factor.

The Alertness System

The alertness system keeps us alert to opportunities and threats in the environment. The alertness system, once activated, reduces reaction time. The attentiveness system, when activated, enables the mind to carry out cognitive tasks including reasoning and remembering. Caffeine stimulates all of the neurotransmitter systems and activates all of the neurons that promote alertness.

Manual Dexterity: A Matter Of Time

Studies have shown that when people who do not use caffeine regularly take large amounts of caffeine, their hand steadiness and manual dexterity are impaired. Recently studies have shown that these impairments may disappear in regular caffeine users over time. Measures of fine motor control, such as tracing images and pegboard tests, on subjects who use caffeine regularly have shown an improvement in these areas.

We mention these effects of caffeine because if you do fine work with your hands you need to be aware that caffeine use may impact your performance.

More on Caffeine in the Workplace

We have already discussed some of the ways that caffeine can improve performance in the workplace. We will take a quick look at a few more examples of this. In addition to increasing wakefulness, alertness, sharpening reasoning, and improving reaction time, caffeine can help eliminate another common workplace problem. Studies have shown that use of caffeine can often relieve these headaches. The result is an overall improvement in workplace efficiency.

A common problem for many in the workplace is a condition known as "Habituation," which quite simply is boredom from repetitious tasks. If you take caffeine before performing repetitive work studies show a dramatic decrease in mistakes, and a commensurate improvement in attitude and productivity. Remember as always to be aware that too much caffeine can work against you.

Games and Caffeine

Games can be great tests of reaction time, logical reasoning, attention, and memory. People tend play them over and over again, which makes for good testing on cognitive performance. Students were tested playing chess, checkers, and bridge.

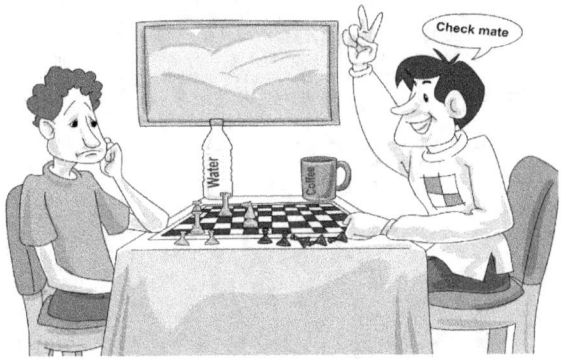

These men and women were tested before and after drinking the equivalent of 150 mg. of caffeine, while playing against the same opponent. The results were striking. The caffeine-supplemented subjects won 1/3 more games than when caffeine-free.

There are no average scores because once again the point for the test is to compare your own score before and after using caffeine. There are a number of other games that you can use to test your performance with and without caffeine.

The Magic That Caffeine Works

Behavioral scientists are diligently working to discover the secret behind caffeine's ability to improve the brain's information processing. There are two popular hypotheses that attempt to explain this power. The first hypothesis attributes caffeine's enhancement of mental functions to a generalized energizing effect. The second hypothesis attributes these enhancements to specific effects on brain and neural activity. There is a third theory that combines both and is perhaps the most complete theory to date attempting to explain the phenomena.

A well known scientist of the 1940s recognized that caffeine acts non-specifically on certain processes concerned with alertness. He also noted caffeine's ability to delay boredom. We know that this idea has been supported by substantial research on the relationship between caffeine and vigilance. He found that caffeine works to refresh a fatigued person, allowing for the enhancing effects of caffeine in the performance of repetitive activity that requires continuous attention.

According to the non-specific energizing theory, caffeine will only improve cognitive performance when a person has become fatigued or bored. The specific cognitive theory believes an improvement will be seen even when a person is rested and alert.

We know that many of caffeine's effects on human performance still remain a mystery to the scientific community. One study shows caffeine helps people repeat numbers, while having an adverse effect on repeating them backward. One study showed caffeine having a positive effect on tests related to speed and cognitive intelligence, but another study suggested that caffeine had a deleterious effect on a given task unless it had been practiced.

It can best be summarized that caffeine gives us beneficial boosts when it comes to performing certain tasks; in others it may interfere with the one's ability to make accurate decisions.

When comparing tests done in a laboratory to real life situations there are many factors to consider. For example one should take into consideration that people choose the jobs they pursue and they are performing tasks for which they have the greatest innate abilities. For one person, programming a computer may be difficult, for another easy. Let's look closer at this example. Caffeine may impair performance for the person having little competency with computer programming. In the person who is competent in programming the use of caffeine will most likely boost performance.

Another important fact to consider is that even for the same person parts of a task may be challenging, while other parts may come more naturally. Caffeine could then actually enhance and impair the same person on different aspects of the same task.

Studies have shown time and again that the more competent you are in performing a task, the more caffeine will help you, and the less able you are the more likely caffeine will impair your efforts.

Caffeine and Short Term Memory

Researchers have recently begun to pay closer attention to the relationship between caffeine and short-term memory. They have found substantial evidence suggesting caffeine improves performance on tasks requiring remembering small amounts of information. They found that caffeine tends to impair or has no effect for tasks requiring subjects to remember a great deal of data.

One recent discovery suggests caffeine causes changes to brain cells. These changes have profound beneficial effects on long-term memory. One way of improving long term memory has to do with the amount of calcium absorbed by brain cells. It is thought caffeine augments the ability of these cells to metabolize calcium.

An experiment was done on the effects of adding caffeine directly to the area of the brain critical for learning and long-term memory. The outcome of the experiment proved that caffeine did indeed increase calcium levels in brain cells.

An even more astonishing affect was that caffeine caused the branching extensions at the end of nerve cells to grow longer, causing new spines and branches to develop. Neuroscientists have long believed that an improvement like this improves both long-term memory and learning.

If these findings can be demonstrated again in future studies, caffeine would be the only substance known that can augment brain functions by altering the physical structure of the brain.

An Unfair Advantage

One scientist has made a valid argument. He argues that if nearly everyone uses caffeine nearly every day, then when a scientist takes a pool of subjects and administers caffeine to one part of the group and withholds it from the others caffeine withdrawal is present in those subjects not receiving caffeine.

He argues that those subjects not receiving caffeine will perform poorly in comparison to those not suffering from withdrawal. If his theory is correct then many of the "improvements" worked by caffeine in psychomotor or cognitive performance may be inaccurate.

A way to avoid this problem is making sure that all the subjects in an experiment have been weaned off of caffeine for at least a week or two before a study is conducted. This way subjects will not be affected by any addiction or withdrawal problems when it comes to caffeine.

Feeling anxious?

Anxiety is the most common psychological disorder in the United States. For some people who have severe anxiety they experience recurring panic attacks. The symptoms of these panic attacks include increased heart rate, palpitations, jitters, irritability, perspiration, and rapid breathing. Caffeine is generally recognized as a substance that can produce anxiety.

One problem is that caffeine binds to adenosine receptors, which interfere with the systems that would otherwise reduce anxiety. Caffeine also interferes with the noradrenergic system, which increases the release of adrenaline. Adrenaline produces a more rapid and stronger heartbeat along with more rapid and deeper breathing. More importantly, adrenaline can produce anxiety. Some studies have shown that when caffeine is combined with emotional distress, there is more adrenaline released than when emotional distress is experienced without caffeine.

One scientist noticed that in countries where anxiety levels tend to be higher people consumed less caffeine in an attempt to avoid aggravating the condition. In countries where caffeine consumption is high anxiety levels tend to be lower.

He also noted that patients with panic disorder have lower caffeine consumption. One study found that when average people were introduced to high levels of caffeine they had panic attacks. Another interesting fact is that the use of anxiety-reducing drugs is higher in people who consume high amounts of caffeine. The question of course is: are people taking more caffeine to combat effects of medications or are they taking medication to counteract the anxiety resulting from high doses of caffeine. Remember it is only in the person who is using caffeine excessively that a correlation with anxiety can be found.

A recent diagnosis has been made that states that caffeine can produce a distinct anxiety disorder. This disorder is beyond any symptoms of anxiety that appear as a normal part of caffeine intoxication and caffeine withdrawal. Caffeine-induced anxiety disorder resembles panic disorder, generalized anxiety disorder, social phobia, and even obsessive-compulsive disorder.

A Lift For Those Feeling Down

Studies have found that some depressive people increase their caffeine consumption in hopes of benefiting more from the euphoric and stimulating power it has.

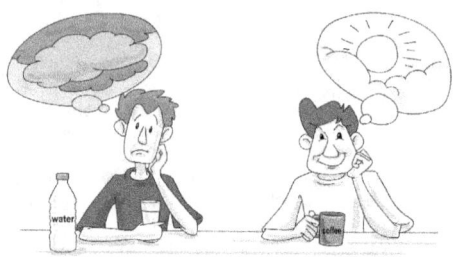

They use caffeine to self-medicate the feelings of despair that often plague them. One study found a strong correlation with depression and high coffee consumption, but only in women.

Another study found that people who consumed at least 200 mg. of caffeine a day tend to have a better disposition than those who didn't. There were even two large scale studies finding that regular coffee drinkers have a lower suicide rate than non-coffee drinkers. In a similar study, the results showed that suicide rate was lower in people who consumed caffeine regardless of the source.

There are those who specialize in depression that argue many of these studies failed to control variables such as the effects of antidepressants and other medications that depressed subjects.

Caffeine and Aggression

There have been recent studies looking at the relationship between caffeine and aggression. Findings suggest that caffeine decreases aggression. It is likely caffeine's ability to inhibit benzodiazepine activity, which is known to increase aggression that lowers aggression in caffeine users. There have been other studies that have contradicted these findings, so this is another area where the true effects of caffeine on human behavior still remain a bit of a mystery.

Caffeine and Rem / Non-Rem Sleep

We have known since the introduction of caffeine that is has the ability to interfere with getting a good night's sleep. There have been studies done finding caffeine to cause insomnia, and other studies showing it causes hypersomnia. Most researchers agree that caffeine can be a real problem when it comes to sleep.

Scientists divide sleep into dreamless sleep and the sleep during which we dream which is referred to as REM sleep. During REM we shift our gaze back and forth following actions in our dreams. Non-REM sleep typically occurs for about an hour before we shift into REM sleep for approximately thirty minutes.

This pattern is repeated throughout the night with non-REM, averaging about 75 percent of our sleep. During non-REM we experience lower heart and respiration rates. During REM sleep there is an increase in heart and respiration rates. Deep muscular relaxation also occurs during REM sleep.

Sleep deficits are caused when any interruption or interference of REM and non-REM sleep occurs. This deficit impairs concentration and diminishes energy throughout the day. The deficit can eventually lead to a higher likelihood of anxiety and depression.

Studies indicate that one out of every three adults experiences sleep disturbances regularly. There are millions of people who take different medications trying to alleviate these disturbances.

There are many factors that affect the way in which caffeine will affect a person's sleep. These include dosage, individual sensitivity to caffeine, and the time between caffeine ingestion and the attempt to sleep. There are many other factors but these three are the most common

One study showed it taking up to four times longer for subjects to fall asleep if they consumed coffee prior to bedtime. Caffeine does more than just lengthen the time it takes to fall asleep, it causes alterations during the onset of REM sleep, total sleep time, and certain characteristics of non-REM sleep. Scientists don't believe that caffeine affects the length of the REM phase of sleep.

However because heavy caffeine users tend to be more restless in bed they experience frequent awakenings and are more likely to be easily awakened. It appears that people are affected differently by caffeine when it comes to sleep.

Studies have shown that based on data collected from people suffering from insomnia there are no reports of high caffeine use among them. High caffeine use is defined as three or more cups of coffee a day. One thing that most studies do agree on is that the closer to bedtime you consume caffeine the higher likelihood it will disrupt your sleep. Sleep disturbances because of caffeine use occur more often in people who are not regular caffeine users.

How caffeine affects sleep according to most research:

1. Caffeine intake near bedtime increases tossing and turning.
2. Caffeine use near bedtime reduces deep sleep and increases light sleep.
3. Caffeine use has no effect on REM sleep.
4. Caffeine use can increase the time it takes to fall asleep up to threefold.
5. Caffeine use can decrease total sleep time by nearly two hours.
6. Caffeine use can increase spontaneous awakenings.

CHAPTER 17 - CAFFEINE INTOXICATION, WITHDRAWAL, & DEPENDENCE

Good communication is as stimulating as black coffee, and just as hard to sleep after. - Anne Morrow Lindbergh

How Much is too Much?

A person would have to consume 100 shots of espresso to reach what is considered a lethal dose of caffeine which is 10 grams. As we know, caffeine can cause physical dependence. We have discussed how upon cessation of use people experience withdrawal symptoms. Caffeine is often characterized by its ability to improve people's moods, self-confidence, and energy. Recently research has shown a pattern of caffeine consumption in some people that merit a diagnosis of clinical dependence syndrome. It is interesting to note that caffeine is the only drug known to support a physical dependence but not a clinical dependence syndrome.

Comparison to lethal drugs of abuse, such as heroin and cocaine, has confused what might otherwise be a relatively straightforward evaluation of the nature and extent of the habit-forming properties of caffeine.

Dependence in the scientific literature is broken down into two classifications: clinical and physical. Physical dependence is where there is withdrawal syndrome after stopping use of a substance. Opium (morphine), cigarettes (nicotine), and coffee (caffeine) fit into this classification. Clinical dependence refers to drugs that can support a clinical dependence. A heroin addict, whose behavior is conditioned by his need to acquire the drug, exhibits a clinical dependence.

Caffeine definitely supports a physical dependence, as shown by the withdrawal symptoms associated with its discontinuation. Drugs that support a clinical dependence syndrome have specific characteristics such as improving people's moods, self-confidence, and energy, and support a desire to constantly get more.

Recently it has been shown that there are people whose amount of caffeine consumption merits a diagnosis of clinical dependence syndrome.

Caffeine Content of Typical Caffeine Drinks

Drink (12 oz)	Mg. of Caffeine
Coffee (6-oz)	130-180
Drip	75-150
Percolated	100
Espresso (1.5 oz)	50-130
Decaf	10-20
Jolt Cola	70
Mountain Dew	54
Diet Mountain Dew	55
Tab	47
Coca-Cola	46
Diet Coke	46
Dr Pepper	40
Diet Dr Pepper	40
Pepsi-Cola	38
Diet Pepsi	36
Canada Dry Diet	1

Symptoms of Caffeine Intoxication

(1) periods of inexhaustibility
(2) rambling speech
(3) flushed face
(4) insomnia
(5) upset stomach
(6) muscle twitching
(7) nervousness
(8) palpitations
(9) restless

The Withdrawal Headache

The caffeine withdrawal headache tends to be more severe when combined with physical exercise. The headache could be easily relieved by consuming more caffeine but that would just start the withdrawal process all over again. In a few days the headaches usually go away. It is only in rare cases that people experience the headache for more than a week.

Patients often report suffering from a caffeine headache when they are not allowed to drink their morning cup of coffee prior to surgery. There are even some doctors who allow patients to get caffeine intravenously to avoid headaches and other withdrawal symptoms during and after operations.

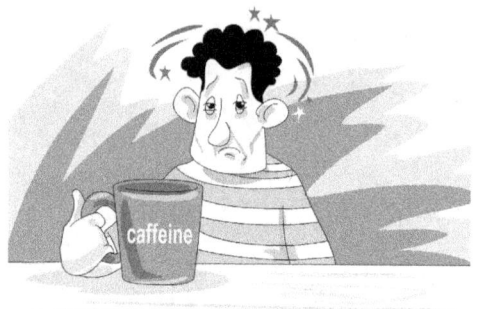

The withdrawal symptoms from caffeine are similar to drugs like heroin. They are flu-like in nature and include; excessive sweating, fatigue, irritability, running nose, and cravings for more caffeine.

One study of newborns who were experiencing withdrawal showed that they were experienced the following symptoms; irritability, jitteriness, and vomiting.

The Question of Clinical Dependence

The scientific community along with psychologists and psychiatrists generally support the idea that caffeine creates a clinical dependence. There is plenty of evidence that supports this idea. Many studies have been done on the issue show that caffeine produces euphoria, energy, and self-confidence. We have previously discussed that caffeine demonstrates a "reinforcing effect" as well. An argument can be made however that these symptoms are far less severe than those found in other widely abused drugs like cocaine.

One question to consider is whether or not people develop a habitual pattern of caffeine use despite any negative consequences they may face. It would appear from many studies done on this issue that there are a small amount of people who do meet this criteria, and therefore it would be permissible to consider caffeine as a drug people can become clinically dependent upon.

Caffeine Intoxication

We know caffeine is the most widely used drug on the planet. We have looked at many areas where caffeine has been linked to different conditions. Here we will take a closer look at the extreme dangers that can come from caffeine intoxication. Generally these problems only occur in people who chronically abuse caffeine.

One study found that many schizophrenics who were observed in the institutional setting were heavy caffeine consumers. A condition known as delirium is linked to extreme caffeine intoxication. People may experience tremors and alterations in levels of consciousness. They will experience high feelings of anxiety along with hallucinations, vertigo, and problems with memory. It is important to note that some of these symptoms may be indirectly linked to caffeine, as insomnia is present in persons experiencing such high levels of caffeine.

Caffeine Poisoning

There is a report of caffeine poisoning dating back to the late 1900s. The reports states the victim suffered from cardiovascular and central nervous system impairments after overdosing on caffeine. There is another report where in the middle of the 20th century a woman died from caffeine overdose. It is interesting to note that many of the cases where caffeine has proved lethal have been when it was administered accidentally by medical personnel.

Medical reports have shown that though it is rare, there are people who have committed suicide by taking lethal doses of caffeine.

There are drugs used by the medical community to counteract the effects of caffeine overdose. The most popular being hem perfusion which flushes the caffeine out of the body. Children can die from a significantly smaller amount of caffeine. One report showed that an infant died from ingesting the equivalent of 3-5 cups of coffee.

Withdrawal

Common symptoms of caffeine withdrawal can include:

1) Sleepiness: drowsiness, yawning
2) Impaired concentration, decreased motivation
3) Irritability, decreased well-being, and self-confidence
4) Reduced friendliness, less talkative
5) Muscle aches and stiffness, nausea or vomiting, blurred vision

Caffeine withdrawal usually begins within twelve to twenty-four hours after stopping caffeine use. It generally peaks within twenty-four to forty-eight hours, and it lasts from about two days to a week. There is great variability both between people and within the same person in the duration and severity of caffeine withdrawal.

Fifty percent of adults, who averaged 3 mg. of caffeine a day, or the equivalent of about two cups of coffee – and did not receive caffeine - had moderate to severe headaches. Ten percent had symptoms of anxiety and depression, and ten percent had significant fatigue.

Caffeine withdrawal can occur after even consuming doses as low as 100 mg. per day, which is the equivalent of about one cup of coffee or two cans of cola.

Eight infants - with suspected caffeine withdrawal - born to mothers who had moderate to heavy caffeine consumption during pregnancies (1,000 mg. a day average). showed symptoms of irritability, jitteriness, and vomiting.

More than eighty percent of all American adults consume caffeine daily, with an average consumption among users of nearly 300 mg. a day. Seventy-five million people would fit the criteria for moderate caffeine clinical dependence.

Reports of caffeine intoxication first appear in medical literature in the middle of the 1800s, and the profile of common symptoms remains unchanged today. The most common are anxiety or nervousness, insomnia, gastrointestinal disturbances, irregular heartbeat, tremors, and psychomotor agitation. Other reported symptoms include excessive urination, headaches, diarrhea, and irregular breathing.

As with any food or drink, caffeine can be a benefit or do harm. Treat it with respect, as a medication, with the ability to change your life for the better.

CHAPTER EIGHTEEN - CAFFEINE IN THE INFORMATION AGE

A mathematician is a machine for turning coffee into theorems. - Paul Erdos

The Universal Appeal

Caffeine will be with us for as long as we can foresee. Caffeine allows us to regulate our thinking and actions so as adjust to the demands of our work and social responsibilities. We can create a 28 hour day or 80 hour work week. We can increase our thinking to keep up with the information age and the speed of computers (at least a little better).

The Future of the Coffeehouse

What role will the coffeehouse of the future play? With its popularity today we can be sure that the coffeehouse will be a viable part of future generations. Caffeine is a

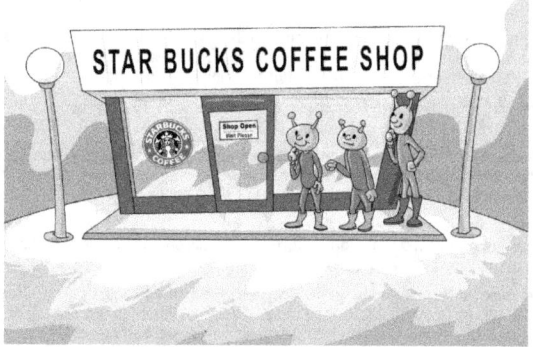

dominant and universally used drug that has become more and more popular as time goes on. We have already seen popular restaurants attempting to compete with coffeehouses by adding specialty coffees and other beverages to their menus.

The coffee bean accounts for the largest international trade of any agricultural product. Nearly every part of the world has been introduced in one way or another to caffeine.

The caffeinated beverage industry is booming and will likely continue to do so into the 22nd century. Consider that the cost of an imported green bean found in coffee is only about 5-8 cents and it is often sold for at least 10 times that amount. Coffeehouses raise prices but people still flock there in droves.

It is a safe bet that in the future the coffeehouse will not only remain viable but will most likely dominate the sidewalks of society even more than it does today.

Caffeine and the Computer

We don't think it's possible to conceive of an internet / bookstore environment with out coffee. Coffee is the socialization medium. Caffeine helps us keep up with the rapid pace of society. Caffeine allows us to multi-task in an age where diverse skills needed to compete on many levels. Coffee is the common ground along with e-mail that allows us to "converse" on the internet on an interplanetary level.

Caffeine the Anti-Oxidant

Caffeine behaves as a "free radical sink," acting as an antioxidant soaking up and neutralizing free radicals. This antioxidant activity of caffeine is similar to the biological antioxidant glutathione. There is a theory that free radicals accumulate in the brain during sleep. According to the theory sleep acts as an antioxidant for the brain. Some studies have shown the antioxidant power of caffeine may be in part responsible for caffeine's revivifying effects.

It is important to note that a lack of activity makes cells more vulnerable to free radical damage; caffeine stimulates brain cells, thereby increase the number and thickness of connections between cells and at the same time preserving those same cells.

Caffeine acts as a blocking agent against free radical activity and actually increases muscle performance as well as protects muscle tissue from damage. Many exercise enthusiasts aren't aware that muscles are the most susceptible tissue to free radical damage. Caffeine can play an important role in sports training because it protects against exercise-induced muscle damage. Caffeine also supplements the body's natural defenses, which is also especially important for anyone who exercises intensely.

Caffeine's Impact on Cellulite

It has been proven that caffeine causes cells to burn fat. Anti-cellulite creams, which have been around since the 17th century, often contain caffeine. Studies have shown that these creams are safe for most people. There was a study done which found that after several weeks a woman lost nearly an inch of cellulite from the thigh when she applied anti-cellulite. Most agree that these types of cream have a significant effect at least temporarily, if not long term. Models often apply such creams before having their pictures taken.

Caffeine and the Fight Against Time

Caffeine has powerful brain-protective and restorative functions. These agents enable caffeine to reduce incidence of degenerative conditions such as Parkinson's disease. Many scientists believe this is true for Alzheimer's as well. Caffeine actually creates a situation where the brain is able to grow new cells in areas responsible for long-term memory. The age-reversing effects of caffeine include improving physical stamina, reasoning, reaction time, motivation, focus, and self-confidence, and memory.

Once we hit middle age we have less motivation to push ourselves physically compared to when we are younger. Motivation can be increases by they psycho-neurological properties in caffeine. Many studies have shown that with proper training people 50 or older can perform as well as those half their age. Caffeine as we know has the ability to lift our mood and this is more apparent in older individuals.

As people age they lose strength, muscle mass, brain cells, bone mass, and the acuteness of the senses. Caffeine works as an effective weapon in the fight against these debilitating ailments because it helps people to exercise harder and longer as well as burn more fat while doing so. It not only speeds up the mind, but thickens dendrites and stimulates axioms to grow. The brain grows on caffeine instead of atrophies.

How Old Are You?

If you think of yourself only in terms of your chronological age, you may quickly become depressed and develop a malaise. But if you consider how hard and long you can work out, how quickly you can think, how well you remember, how good your sex life is, how excited you are about work and life, then you may and should consider yourself as "young as you feel."

Caffeine and Pain

Caffeine alleviates pain by blocking a nerve's its ability to signal pain. In addition, caffeine stimulates the body's own painkilling mechanism. Caffeine changes the way pain signals are dealt with. Caffeine restores the balance of the serotonin system, and thereby relieves migraines and acts as a mood boost. Caffeine has a positive effect on lowering pain sensitivity and magnifies our sense perceptions, so we perceive more enjoyment in life.

A Final Word

Caffeine is to be enjoyed not abused. It in many ways is a medication that can be very dangerous if overindulged in. As we know, drinking too much of any caffeinated beverage can cause you to get nauseous, anxious, and confused. When you experience these negative side effects you will most likely stop drinking any caffeinated beverages, which means you will not experience any of the many benefits caffeine has to offer when properly used. Remember more is not better! We wish you good luck? I believe luck is for the unprepared so rather we wish you success, which can be guaranteed if you follow the steps we have laid out for you.

APPENDIX "A" - THE SIX NEWEST FAT-BURNING INGREDIENTS

Don't like coffee? Caffeine makes you nervous? No problem! We've found a solution! Check out these six supplements, and know that we've found an answer for everyone. Since ephedra was taken off the market, people have been looking for a worthy fat-burning replacement. Well, here are the newest, cutting edge supplements.

1) Aspidosperma quebracho-blanco (AQB). This is a South American evergreen tree species. The bark contains several alkaloids that act as central-nervous system stimulators that can help you get lean. Dosage: 50-250 mgs. Of AQB extract standardized for .3% alkaloids taken twice daily.

2) Sesamin. This is a lignan from sesame oil. The active ingredient turns on genes that increase fat oxidation and decrease fat storage. Dosage: 500-1000 mg. of sesamin 2-3 times a day with food.

3) Hops Extract. New research reports that isomerized hops extract can decrease body fat by inhibiting the absorption of fat by the intestines. Secondly, it activates genes involved in fat oxidation to ramp up fat burning. Thirdly, it decreases the activity of genes that control storage of body fat. Dosage: 200-400 mg. of hops extract 1-3 times a day.

4) Oleoylethanol-Amide (OEA). When you eat a meal, the production of OEA increases and woks to ramp up fat-burning and decrease fat storage. Users say it decreases hunger. When you take extra OEA, you essentially trick your body into thinking you've already eaten. OEA is a non-stimulating appetite suppressant and fat burner. Dosage: 25-50 mg of OEA twice a day with food.

5) Tetradecylthioacetci acid (TTA). TTA is specialized fatty acid that regulates the burning and storage of dietary fats. TTA helps decrease LDL and total cholesterol levels and boosts insulin sensitivity. Dosage: 1000 mg. of TTA twice daily

6) Inula Racemosa. This is an herb that grows in the Himalayas. Their roots contain lactones that give it medicinal properties. The most important of these is alantolactone, which enhances insulin sensitivity; meaning you secrete less insulin after eating and less of the meal is stored as dietary fat. Dosage: as per label on Hydroxycut Hardcore.

APPENDIX "B" - THE BEST SWEETENER IN THE WORLD

Naturolose is our brand name for tagatose, a naturally occurring ketose that is found in some dairy products and other foods. We have patented the use of it as a low-calorie, full-bulk sweetener, and also the process to make it starting from whey, a dairy by-product. Naturolose has been determined to be a Generally Recognized As Safe (GRAS) substance in the U.S., with the FDA permitting its use in foods and beverages. Naturolose has also been determined GRAS for use in cosmetics and toothpastes, and in drugs.
Naturolose can currently be used as a sweetener in toothpaste, mouthwash, and other cosmetics, and can also be used as an excipient (non-active ingredient) in over-the-counter and prescription medications.

Naturolose Quick Facts

1) The taste of sugar – far better than any low-calorie sweetener. Taste tests show that you can't tell the difference between Naturolose and table sugar.
2) No aftertaste like some other bulk sweeteners or high intensity sweeteners.
3) Naturolose is 92% as sweet as table sugar.
4) Unlike other sweeteners that require special tricks for baking, Naturolose browns and bakes.
5) Naturolose has anti-plaque, anti-biofilm, anti-halitosis, and non-cariogenic properties. It does not cause cavities and does not promote tooth decay – so dentists encourage its use.
6) Naturolose doesn't cause glucose spikes, so no sugar rush or sugar crash occurs
7) Naturolose is a prebiotic – promoting general gut health by promoting healthy bacteria and inhibiting dangerous ones.

Benefits Of Naturolose

1) Weight Loss at Healthy Rate
2) Diabetes (safe and beneficial for diabetics)
3) Anti-hyperglycemic
4) Anti-plaque, Non-cariogenic, and Anti-halitosis
5) Prebiotic
6) Fights Colon Cancer
7) Anti-Biofilm
8) Increases Beneficial HDL-cholesterol

Naturolose & Obesity

According to the American Obesity Association , approximately 127 million adults in the U.S. are overweight, 60 million obese, and 9 million severely obese. Obesity is linked to the following diseases: high blood pressure, type 2 diabetes, heart disease, stroke, gall bladder disease and cancer of the breast, prostate and colon.

Naturolose can become a vital tool in the fight against obesity. Studies show that Naturolose promotes weight loss when incorporated into a routine diet. Human clinical trials conducted on patients with type 2 diabetes and normal persons at the Department of Endocrinology at the University of Maryland School of Medicine showed that both the type 2 diabetics and normal subjects receiving the daily regimen of Naturolose (tagatose) for 12 months, gradually and consistently lost weight at medically desirable rates. BioSpherix is in the process of investigating Naturolose in various products and formulations to combat weight gain and diseases connected to obesity.

APPENDIX "C" CAFFEINE CONTENT AND WEIGHT EQUIVALENCIES

6 ounce cup of instant coffee	I 00 mg.
6 ounce cup filter drip coffee	150 mg.
8 ounce cup filter drip coffee	200 mg.
Thermo Power Boost® tablet	100 mg.

Bodyweight equivalencies

1.5 mg. per kilogram = 65 mg. for 100 pound person
3.0 mg. per kilogram = 130 mg. for 100 pound person
4.5 mg. per kilogram = 200 mg. for 100 pound person
1.5 mg. per kilogram = 100 mg. for 150 pound person
3.0 mg. per kilogram = 200 mg. for 150 pound person
4.5 mg. per kilogram = 300 mg. for 150 pound person
1.5 mg. per kilogram = 130 mg. for 200 pound person
3.0 mg. per kilogram = 260 mg. for 200 pound person
4.5 mg. per kilogram = 400 mg. for 200 pound person

Amounts of Caffeine Equivalent to 150 mg. for a 150 Pound Person

100 lbs. (45 kg)	100 mg	4 oz.
120 lbs. (54 kg)	120 mg	5 oz.
150 lbs. (67.5 kg)	150 mg	6 oz.
175lbs. (79 kg)	175 mg	7 oz.
200 lbs. (90 kg)	200 mg	8 oz.
250 lbs. (1I2.5 kg)	250 mg	10 oz.
300 lbs. (135 kg)	300 mg	12 oz.

Sources And Dosages Of Caffeine

Caffeine is not like other drugs that require increasingly greater amounts to achieve the previous results. Caffeine requires about fifteen minutes to enter the system and begin working. But take note. When caffeine is combined with carbohydrates – the sugar you dump in – the majority of caffeine's effects of fat-burning potential is blunted because of the subsequent rise in the fat-storing hormone insulin. The effects of caffeine usually last three to four hours. The effective dosage varies greatly from person to person – anywhere from 50 to 500 mgs. Start with 50 mg. and increasing the dose until you experience the benefits without the side effects. Following are a number of sources of caffeine and their content:

Source	Caffeine (mg.)
Coffee, drip, 6 oz.	80-175
Coffee, instant, 6 oz	60-I00
Coffee, decaffeinated, 6 oz	2-5
Tea, 5-minute steep, 6 0z.	20-100

APPENDIX "D"- CALCULATING YOUR BODY MASS INDEX

A healthy weight goes beyond the number on the scale: There's also your body mass index (BMI), which is a measurement that determines if you're at an appropriate weight for your height by estimating your <u>body fat</u>. To calculate your BMI, your height and weight are entered into a mathematical equation and the resulting number reveals whether you're underweight, normal weight, overweight or obese.

Though BMI is generally a reliable approximation of body fat, it doesn't always tell the whole picture. "BMI doesn't differentiate between body fat and lean muscle mass," says Wayne Westcott, Ph.D., fitness research director at the South Shore YMCA in Quincy, Mass. and author of several books on fitness. BMI might be a poor indicator of body fat in athletes, people who have a muscular build and those who are heavily engaged in strength training because their dense muscle mass may classify them as overweight when they aren't. On the flip side, it might underestimate body fat in older individuals and people who have lost muscle mass.

Even with its drawbacks, however, BMI can give you a rough idea of how healthy you are. "You can use BMI to help you evaluate whether you need to make lifestyle changes," Westcott says.

You can determine your BMI by using a <u>calculator,</u> where you'll be asked to plug in your height and weight. Or you can figure out your BMI with this formula:
(Weight in pounds) divided by [(height in inches) x (height in inches)] x 703. Once you've determined your BMI, use the following chart to determine where you fit in:

Below 18.5:	Underweight
18.5 - 24.9:	Normal
25 - 29.9:	Overweight
30 and above:	Obese

If your BMI is 25 or above and you're not an athlete or you don't have a muscular build, you could be at risk for numerous health conditions including heart disease, type 2 diabetes. Talk with your physician about losing weight. On the other hand, if you're underweight, consult with your physician to determine if and how you should gain weight. For women, being underweight can interrupt the menstrual cycle and cause bone loss.

COPYRIGHT

J.W. Enterprises
3595 Hayden Pl. Suite One
Boulder, CO 80301

Printed by CreateSpace, an Amazon.com company
CreateSpace, Charleston, SC

Available from Amazon and other online stores.
Available on Kindle and other devices.

Graphic Art by izueyes777

JOIN THE FIGHT

Thank you for believing in me and the Why We Eat program.

Please go to: whyweeat.com (then "blogs") to read all my timely articles on diet, nutrition and the latest scientific discoveries.

And you can sign up for notices of upcoming books by going to "contact me.")

(I promise not to share your email with anyone else, and I won't clutter your inbox.   I'll only contact you when a new book is out).

If you loved the book, and have a moment to spare, a positive review on Amazon would be much appreciated and help to get "the word" out.

It's simple: go back on line to where you purchased or saw the book on Amazon. Click on the image of the book. Scroll down the page until you come to "Customer reviews." Then "write a review." I'm hoping you feel strongly enough to choose "5 Stars."

ABOUT THE AUTHOR

I attended Drexel University (B.S.), Temple University (M.B.A.) The University of Pennsylvania (M.A.), and Clayton College (Ph.D., Naturopathic Medicine) - where I gained unique insights in the realm of health and nutrition.

In regard to obesity and diet, I have corresponded with the health ministries of Australia, Mexico, The United Kingdom, the new health director of he European Union, and the U.S. Secretary of Health And Human Services concerning my work in the field of nutrition.

I have developed a food tax that he presented to appropriate members of the U.S. Senate, where it has received serious attention. I have created a statistical protocol that takes into account personal choices in determining appropriate individual costs for Medicare and Medicaid. These programs fall under an umbrella I have labeled Vested Interest and Economic Incentive.

On an individual basis, I have counseled hundreds of people - working with ailments as diverse as obesity, Alzheimer's, Parkinson's, CFS, ADD, Multiple Sclerosis, liver disease, numerous forms of cancer, and diabetes.

I have advised school districts on alternative methodologies in dealing with their lunch programs. I am on the board of directors for Insulite Labs: a leader in PCOS research and development.

I have consulted with Markos Kyprianou, Health Commission for the European Union, which includes 6 countries with obesity rates higher than the U.S.

My work on obesity has been recognized by the office of the President of Mexico and is being used to implement programs to combat obesity in that country.

And now I have the opportunity to help millions of individuals who have failed over and over in their efforts to control their weight, and to this moment had all but given up hope.

ACKNOWLEDGEMENTS

I would like to thank my parents for surrounding me with books at an early age, encouraging me to read, and explore, and to challenge conventional wisdom. To Tim Rea for his unwavering inspiration and direction. And to my brother, Michael Weiss, who has overcome adversity far greater than I will ever be challenged by. His example led me to believe in my work and myself when, at times, the effort seemed beyond my capabilities, and without whose love this book would never have been completed.

DISCLAIMER

The information in this book is based on the latest scientific research. However, before you embark on your new path, consult of a qualified physician to ascertain your basic health. The best practitioners and the best programs are those that combine the knowledge of allopathic and naturopathic medicine.

There are many well-meaning health care professionals working hard to assist people in their struggles with their weight and health issues. However, doctors, nurses, and dieticians, are trained in conventional medicine. This is the age of specificity: where people get paid more and more for knowing less and less. Diet, nutrition, and exercise all affect ones ability to overcome their weight issues. No one discipline will succeed in overcoming all the obstacles and attaining ones goals.

WHAT'S NEXT

Look for the fourth book in the Why We Eat series, "Turning off the Hunger Gene: food as medicine in the 21st century: coming in 30 days to Amazon. Following is the synopsis…

TURNING OFF THE HUNGER GENE: FOOD AS MEDICINE IN THE 21ST CENTURY

Until now, no one has been able to tell you why weight loss programs do not work. Why you can lose weight at first, but then becomes impossible to keep it off. Why 95% of us who go on a diet fail, and over 50% actually weigh more at the end of a program than they did at the beginning. Well, after thirty years of research, I have found the answer.

The neurobiology of eating starts when signals from the mouth flow through the nerves to the brain. Dopamine, and opioids (endorphin-like biochemicals) then flow, creating a sense of pleasure. At the same time, hormones are released that begin to either curb the appetite or stimulate it, depending upon which foods we choose.

The process of eating relies upon a vast array of circuitry between the brain and the stomach and small intestines. Our brains are effectively linked to our gut by the hypothalamus, the brain structure that is the control center for weight regulation. The stomach and intestines produce hormones that activate the hypothalamus, and neurons in the hypothalamus then send new messages back to the body.

Some foods, when ingested, quickly send signals to the brain telling us that we are full. However, many of the foods we consume today have the opposite effect – muting the "full" signal to the brain, stimulating the appetite control center, and encouraging us to keep eating.

Saturated and polyunsaturated fats (which are even worse for you) give food the texture, aromas, and tastes that trigger the appetite by an evolutionary process. The smells of processed foods set off sets off an endorphin reaction that signals the brain to crave food and binge.

Endorphins are biochemicals in the body that are hundreds of times stronger than morphine or opiates and bring on a sense of euphoria. In experiments, when given a choice, mice and chimps chose endorphins over food and sex.

It does no good to know which foods are good for you if you can't control your runaway appetite. Further, what good is exercise when it takes 8 ½ hours of walking at a brisk pace to work off the calories from one fast food meal?

The purveyors of magic elixirs, severely restricted calorie diets, blood type diets, low-carb diets, high-protein diets have no clue as to why people are always hungry. Their advice and findings are based on limited research and faulty logic.

The manufacturers and sellers of fast foods infuse their foods with chemicals that increase the appetite and create habitual use just like tobacco or other drugs. Our water is cleansed with Aluminum Chloride which affects the thyroid and slows down the metabolism, making it almost impossible to lose weight and keep it off. It seems as though all the forces of science work against us when it comes to gaining / losing weight. Well, we're going to use science to fight back. And our science is newer and more powerful than theirs. We are going to win this battle.

With *Turning off the Hunger Gene* you will regain control of your appetite and choose foods that are best for you, not the most tempting. You will reach not only your weight goals, but your life goals as well.